LOSING, LEARNING, AND LOVING

Through Christ's example, learn how contestants
on a reality weight-loss show achieve wellness
by healing body, mind, and soul

KELLY CP HUDSON, MS, ATC

Losing, Learning, and Loving
Copyright © 2021 by Kelly CP Hudson

Cover Design and Artwork by: 100 Covers
Formatted by: Cutting Edge Studio

No contestants were harmed during the filming of the show, however, we did shrink them significantly.

DEDICATION

This book is dedicated to the people who gave me permission
to live courageously and write this book.

My father-in-law, Bill Hudson, has encouraged me for many years
to write a book. "Geez, Kelly, ya got a book there!"

AND

Fr. Daniel Barica, OFM. He too saw a book within me
and challenged me to finally put pen to paper.

While I was writing this book, both men were diagnosed with
cancer. Please join me in praying for their healing and recovery.

And most especially this book is dedicated to
the three seasons of contestants that have made
me a better athletic trainer, wife, mother, and woman of God.
It has been an honor and privilege to serve you,
contribute to your wellness journey, and to now call you my friends.

Table of Contents

PREMIERE

I was scheduled to speak at a women's conference being held in a local church in just a few weeks and hadn't yet chosen a topic. I could usually come up with something to talk about, even in a pinch. After all, I am a full-blooded Irish girl, and storytelling seems almost second nature. But I was completely out of stories. It was a "gabbers" block like I had never experienced. I can't say my husband wasn't happy. He'd been waiting for me to hit a word block for years. I felt like I was running out of time, and as the weeks crept closer, I was sure I'd have to call and cancel for lack of content. But as Zig Ziglar says: "Lack of direction, not lack of time, is the problem. We all have twenty-four hour days."

So I got out my compass and chose a direction. For years, I had toyed with the idea of introducing a self-improvement guide focusing on how the body, mind, and soul are woven together to create the elusive state referred to as wellness. But the intention was all I had, and I was struggling to relate it to my current professional position, which was why I was asked to speak at the conference in the first place. I'll tell you more about that as we get better acquainted.

Then it happened. I was sitting in Mass dreading that I had to go home and get started on this lecture with nothing more than an idea. Then I remembered that there was someone who could help me; in fact, I was in His house. So I took a deep breath, swallowed my pride, and asked God to take the wheel.

Following my plea, the Gospel reading that day, John 8:1–11—the story of the woman accused—hit me like a ton of stones (so to speak), and the presentation practically prepared itself. The words came together, and the stories emerged one after another. Not to be overly dramatic, but it was as if I was blessed with the gift of tongues, if that gift had been for witty anecdotes and sensational stories. I was seeing what I had always known but rarely submitted to: When you ask God for help, He delivers. But He does it bigger and better than you could possibly imagine. So, I have since taken what I discovered in the Gospel reading that day and married it to my idea of presenting on wellness and how healing of body, mind, and soul are the instructions to being well.

For years, I have spoken this message to groups all over Orange and Los Angeles counties, but I really wanted to share these simple life-changing lessons with more people, so again I turned to God for a little assistance. But as I'm reminded, God doesn't deal in little; He always goes above and beyond what you can imagine is possible. When I asked Him for help with getting this message to more ears, He said, "Get a good pen!" So here I am, with God's blessing, a speaker trying to be a writer. That might help you understand why I use an overabundance of exclamation points.

Our hope, mine and God's (I feel at liberty to speak for Him since we are partners in this book), is that the information being presented will encourage you to seek healing in the areas of your life that need it most. And that through this healing, you will discover true wellness and live your life abundantly.

I've never been a fan of lengthy introductions. I usually just want to get to the good stuff. So what are we waiting for? Grab yourself a soothing spot of tea, an energizing cup of joe, or a heavenly hot toddy if that suits you, then invite God to join you as you discover how losing, learning, and loving has changed the lives of the most courageous people I know. And how renewing your own body, mind, and soul will enable you to reconcile the things that have been holding you back and will allow you to transform your life.

God speed ahead!

Season 1

HEALING

The Woman's Story

Picture, if you will, the following scene:

In the town's central gathering place, an angry crowd had assembled because on that particular day, a sinner had been exposed, and the law of the moral guardians needed to be upheld.

Leading the mob were the righteous and indignant, those who hadn't been caught breaking the law. They were on the ready to cast —judgement, to chastise, and to pity the recipient of this "well-deserved" punishment.

In the center of the angry horde stood the victim whose weeping eyes were cast downward in the utmost of shame, for sins of the body had been completely and utterly exposed. With a body abused, a mind littered with lies, and a soul aching for peace, the outcast of society cowered, defenseless and humiliated, desperate to change anything and everything.

Now, you might assume the scene I'm setting up is from the well-known biblical story of the woman accused and the onlookers who were ready to stone her for her sins. But the events I'm detailing actually hit a bit closer to home. This scene plays out each and every day that I go to work. You see... I work in reality TV.

For the last three seasons of *The Biggest Loser*, I served as the head athletic trainer, and most recently, director of sports medicine. In the three seasons that I spent on the show, I was blessed to meet some of the most determined and courageous people this world has to offer. People who were desperately searching for something better for themselves and their families. So what does this have to do with the scene above? As you will soon see, a great deal.

While I was working on the show, I couldn't help but notice the unmistakable parallels between the woman in the story who was clearly an outcast of society and the way our cast members had been made to feel by the world, as they struggled to get their weight under control. But even more alarming was the resemblance that I saw between those casting judgement with... well, to be completely honest, us, the viewing public.

You see, each and every season our cast members are desperate for change. They know that they have not been living their true potential and are not presenting the world with the best they have to offer. They know that their current lifestyle is subject to ridicule and disdain. But, like most of us, they also know that making a drastic life change is easier said than done. They understand that, while on this journey, they will have to confront physical pain, mental anguish, and a whole slew of judgement for the state of their bodies, based on society's perceptions of overeating and laziness.

In front of us, their audience and their judge, they will stand remorseful and humiliated, with the "sins" committed against their bodies completely and utterly exposed. Their minds are filled with lies about themselves and what they are capable of achieving, and their souls are broken and in desperate need of healing.

Essentially, they are in need of wellness, just like the woman who was caught in the act of adultery. In John's beautiful biblical story of renewal, Jesus shows us how healing, creating wholeness, and experiencing wellness are possible. Let me show you what I mean. We have already set up the scene, so let's take it from there with the Gospel of John 8:4–11:

> "Teacher, this woman has been caught in the act of adultery. Now in the law Moses commanded us to stone such. What do you say about her?" This they said to test him, that they might have some charge to bring against

him. Jesus bent down and wrote with his finger on the ground. And as they continued to ask him, he stood up and said to them, "Let him who is without sin among you be the first to throw a stone at her." And once more he bent down and wrote with his finger on the ground. But when they heard it, they went away, one by one, beginning with the eldest, and Jesus was left alone with the woman standing before him. Jesus looked up and said to her, "Woman, where are they? Has no one condemned you?" She said, "No one, Lord." And Jesus said, "Neither do I condemn you; go, and do not sin again."

Jesus addresses healing in three critical areas of this woman's life in order for her to be whole or well. Let's break it down.

Jesus first heals her mind by changing how she views herself. Jesus asks, "Woman, where are they? Has no one condemned you?" Jesus clearly knows the answer to this question, as He is the one that sent them all away. Then He does something incredible: He allows the woman to voice the answer. To which she responds, "No one, Lord." He does this because there is incredible power in our own self-talk, how we view ourselves, and the world around us. This woman is, maybe for the first time in her life, allowed to say, and truly believe, "There is no one here to hurt me. I am no longer a victim. I am strong enough to walk away." When we see that Jesus loves us, we can begin to love ourselves, and we are no longer the victim of our own self-destructive behaviors. We become bold in His love.

But Jesus isn't done yet. He then sets out to heal her soul. Notice that the woman refers to the stranger that saved her as Lord. Because she recognizes Him as the Lord, He heals her soul. He frees her of the guilt, shame, and pain she has carried with her for a lifetime by offering her these words: "Neither do I condemn you." Her soul is then set free. When we recognize Christ in our lives, He offers to free us from the guilt, shame, and pain that we are carrying. With His generous mercy, He redeems our souls.

Jesus lastly addressed the abuse of her body by telling her, "Go, and do not sin again." The wounds you inflict on your flesh are sinful because God has given you a body in which the Holy Spirit resides. With these words, He is telling her to heal the physical wounds and encourages her to go back into the world and use her body in virtuous ways—ways that will honor God. We are called to honor the physical body that God has gifted to us by keeping it in check, because through our healthy body, we bring God's love to the world.

In order for the woman to fully heal, to be whole, and to experience wellness, Jesus shows her that she will have to grow and change in these three critical areas of her life: body, mind, and soul.

> *May the God of peace himself sanctify you wholly; and may your spirit and soul and body be kept sound and blameless at the coming of our Lord Jesus Christ.*
> *—1 Thessalonians 5:23*

Well, Well, Well

You see, wellness is an integration of body, mind, and soul. It is the awareness that every thought we have, emotion we feel, and action we take, along with every word we express, belief we hold, and value we profess, impacts our overall state of health. Wellness is so much bigger than simply being free of illness.

The World Health Organization defines wellness "as a state of complete physical, mental, and social well-being, and not merely the absence of disease or infirmity." [i]

The National Wellness Institute agrees that wellness is a conscious, self-directed, and evolving process of achieving full potential and therefore defines wellness as "an active process through which people become aware of, and make choices toward, a more successful existence." [ii]

The Wellness Council of America states that "wellness is the active pursuit to understand and fulfill your individual human needs—which allows you to reach a state where you are flourishing and able to realize your full potential in all aspects of life." [iii]

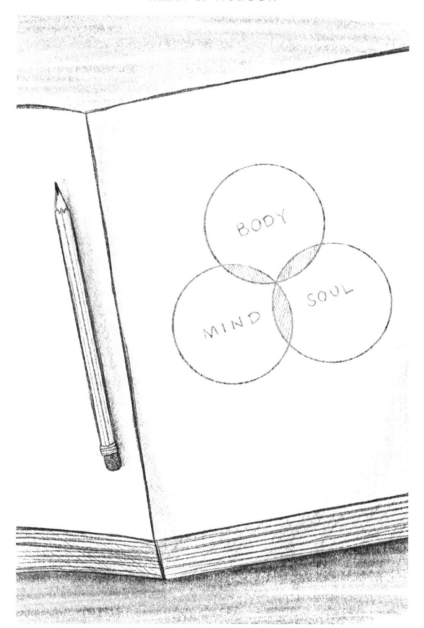

The Global Wellness Institute (GWI) defines wellness as the active pursuit of activities, choices, and lifestyles that lead to a state of holistic health (the health of the whole person). [iv]

Incidentally, in May 2020, as a result of the COVID-19 pandemic, the GWI announced a collaborative effort with the Vatican focused on "resetting the world with wellness." Both the Pope and the GWI believe that wellness can provide a roadmap for not only individuals but also for world healing and growth.[v]

With each of these definitions, you can easily see that wellness is so much more than just being free from illness. Wellness is a dynamic process of change and growth that can lead us to live our very best lives.

Sounds good, doesn't it? So how do you and I achieve wellness? Where do we start?

Well, let's start with what we know. God loves our human bodies. He created our bodies to reveal His love to us. Ironically, I am in the middle of a hot flash as I write this sentence, so I understand if you are thinking, My God, my God, why have you abandoned me with this broken down, outdated model? Or, seriously, God, you couldn't spring for the newer, easier to care for edition? There are definitely times that we all feel that way. But stick with me here.

In *Theology of the Body*, St. John Paul II writes about the body[vi]:

> *The body, in fact, and only the body, is capable of making visible what is invisible: the spiritual and the divine. It was created to transfer into the visible reality of the world the mystery hidden from eternity in God and thus to be a sign of it.*
> —TOB 19:4

The human body reveals the mystery of God's love for human beings. Therefore, we are charged with the upkeep of this incredibly important gift. Wow! That's a lot of responsibility, huh? But don't be discouraged. Much like everything God grants us, He also provides us with exactly what we need to handle it. It's one of my favorite things about Him! We just need to look to Him for the instructions. So let's stop living in fear and start operating from a place of faith, because that is when we will begin to see a difference in our lives.

Stay Tuned

Before we get too far, this seems like a prime time to make sure you are dialed in with the layout of the book. In place of standard sections, chapters, and conclusions you will find seasons, episodes, and finales to guide you through the stories of various Biggest Loser contestants and their wellness journeys.

At the end of each episode, you will find a segment entitled "Weighing In": this is where former contestants, other industry professionals that have worked on the show, and I (when I've had an afterthought) "weigh in" on the subject. There we'll offer additional suggestions, encouragement, and resources so you can get started in that particular area of healing, change, and growth to begin your own wellness journey.

One last important note. Please remember that this book is not about losing weight; it is about healing the whole person—body, mind, and soul—through the strength of the Lord so you can be the best possible you, because only then do you reflect God Himself. So don't touch that dial and enjoy the show!

Season 2

BODY

Megan's Story

"Do you not know that your body is a temple of the Holy Spirit within you, which you have from God? You are not your own; you were bought with a price. So glorify God in your body."
—1 Corinthians 6:19–20

Megan, a gorgeous young woman, was pursuing her dream career in the fitness industry and regularly moonlighted as a plus-size model. Unfortunately, even though she was excellent at her job, she was told by her superiors that she would never be promoted in the the fitness world due to her weight. So she worked even harder to prove that she was an exceptional employee. She took on additional assignments and went the extra mile just to prove her worth in the company. But since she was putting so much of herself into her job, she was completely depleted of time and energy to care for the things that really mattered, including her own health. She was eating poorly, often dehydrated, and was no stranger to sleepless nights. And although she spent a great deal of time in fitness centers, she wasn't making it a priority to exercise herself. She was doing everything in her power to advance her career but her work ethic was taking a physical toll. Until finally one day she realized that those in charge were never going to see her the way she saw herself, a competent, hard-working employee; they were only going to see her weight. For Megan, physical health had at one time been a huge priority, but life and ironically a career in fitness were putting it on a back burner, and the results of it were catching up to her—not only in her professional life but her personal life as well. She was living the perfect storm of unhealthy, and her body was clearly affected by the bad habits that had become routine in her life.

Megan needed to make some major changes. But where do you start when you realize that your current lifestyle is wreaking havoc on your physical body? How about on a reality TV show? So Megan auditioned for *The Biggest Loser*. Her compelling story and bubbly personality easily earned her a spot on the twelve-person cast that appeared in the 2020 reboot of the show.

With the help of her Biggest Loser support team, Megan was able to answer the question, "Where do I start?" And she learned that in order to make big changes in her life, she would have to go back to the basics. Even Dr. Seuss reminds us that "sometimes the questions are complicated and the answers simple."

Remember that the human body was designed to thrive because it's through our bodies that God works in our lives and makes a difference in the world. So in order for our bodies to flourish, we have to address the four main components of physical health. They are the fundamentals of the human body, and by addressing each of these components, we start the groundwork from which we can build a sustainable and healthy lifestyle. Laying an unshakable foundation begins with:

- Exercise
- Nutrition
- Hydration
- Recovery

Now if you have ever seen *The Biggest Loser*, you know that we always start our contestants in the gym with our iconic first chance workout. And the reason we always start in the gym while on the road to physical health is because simply adding more activity to your life provides countless benefits. However, if the very thought of increasing your physical activity makes you sweat, think about this... wouldn't any of us fix up our home if the Pope was spending the night?

Of course we would because something Holy would be residing

inside. (And my dear mother would be so embarrassed if I didn't!) The home that God has chosen is within each of us; within our very own bodies holiness resides. Therefore, we are charged with its maintenance and upkeep. Exercise is a proven way to keep our bodies in tip-top shape, both inside and out. So grab your Bible, and let's head over to the gym.

A Bible at the gym? Don't worry. We aren't using it for step-ups or deadlifts... although a Bible boot camp isn't a half-bad idea. Next book!

Episode 1:

EXERCISE

Whenever I attempt a new skill, experiment in the kitchen, or take a trip to parts unknown, I like to have some type of a guide, directions, or a roadmap. Certainly, taking care of your body is no different. A guide will assure that you are headed in the correct direction and will right you when you go astray. When our contestants arrive at the gym, they are gifted with personal trainers to lead them on their fitness journey and to gently (and sometimes not so gently) guide them back when they go off course, reminding them why they are there and how capable they are of success.

Any ideas where you can find that type of guidance and support? Here's a hint: You carried it into the gym with you. That's right, the Bible. As you will see throughout this book, the Holy Bible is a phenomenal resource overflowing with pearls of wisdom regarding the care of God's greatest creation, you and me! What you won't find in there is the latest fad diet or a discounted membership to the gym. But what you will find is evidence that God loves our bodies and wants us to care for them, along with reasons to carry on and encouragement to stay the course.

So let's see what the Bible has to say about exercise.

If you remember from the New Testament, St. Paul wrote letters to Timothy to guide and assist him on his mission to shepherd a congregation of early Christians. Paul counsels Timothy on various ways to care for his flock and for himself as he labors in setting up the church. In one of my favorite verses, Paul mentions physical training:

For while bodily training is of some value, godliness is of value in every way, as it holds promise for the present life and also for the life to come.
—1 Timothy 4:8

Paul seems to be saying that bodily training is of limited value compared to godliness, which has value in all things. But I like to think with everything we know now, that even in the early days of Christianity, they preached that physical fitness was of some value because our bodies are of great value. And that in order to do God's work successfully, we need to be in good physical condition. In addition, training our bodies takes effort, tenacity, and discipline, strengths that will benefit us in all aspects of life, especially our spiritual life. The gym is a great place to master those skills. Lastly, I'm intrigued by the idea that even in 100 AD, athletic trainers would have been able to find work! Where people are physically active, athletic trainers are always busy.

Now, in full disclosure, I should also mention that, only a few chapters later, Paul advises Timothy to stop drinking so much water and to have a little wine! So... I guess we should take all of his fitness advice with a grain of salt and just remember the old saying "fitness is next to godliness." I think that's how it goes!

Nonetheless, the point remains. There is value in taking care of our physical bodies, especially when we are setting out to do the Lord's work. And, apparently, a glass of wine now and again is St. Paul approved.

So let's talk about why bodily training is of value. Here are just a few of the ways that exercise and activity benefit us all:

- Reduces risk of heart disease and stroke
- Reduces risk of some cancers
- Decreases blood pressure*
- Decreases risk of diabetes*
- Decreases back pain
- Creates stronger bones and muscles

- Increases balance and decreases the likelihood of falling
- Increases energy levels
- Increases self-esteem
- Puts you in a better mood because activity fights depression and reduces stress
- Reduces the risk of dementia and increases brain power
- Promotes better sleep
- Helps you control your weight

*We see notable, positive changes in our contestants' blood pressure and diabetic status within weeks of starting a regular exercise program.

With all that to gain, it's no wonder we start every season with a first chance workout.

But if you don't have a personal trainer at your side whipping you into shape, you might not know where to begin. With all of the infomercials, gym choices, and exercise equipment on the market, physical fitness can seem daunting, especially if someone is just getting started. But don't be discouraged. I'll show you how easily you can make physical activity a part of your daily life and start reaping all the benefits it has to offer.

Let's get physical

Remember that on *The Biggest Loser*, we take people who have been sedentary for decades and get them into the gym and moving on the first day they arrive. (Important note: I only recommend this strategy with medical support and supervision. Always check with your doctor prior to starting any fitness program.) If they can do it, you can do it. The trick is to not let the idea of exercise overwhelm you, and instead, just simply add more movement into your life.

For instance, if you find yourself driving around a parking lot praying to the patron saint of open parking spots (which, incidentally, may be my husband's grandmother, Grandma O'Brien), you have an opportunity to add movement into your life. So park your car in the farthest space (you know they're always available) and take a stroll. No equipment needed, and you have exercised!

Take the stairs instead of the lazy-vator whenever possible. You didn't even have to sign up for a class, and you have squeezed exercise into your day.

Do you sit at a desk all day? Use your breaks to get up and go! Change your office chair out for an exercise ball for part of the day, or prop your computer to create a standing desk. Set an alarm and experiment with some type of movement every two hours. Just a few minutes are all you need.

If you have kids, you have physical fitness at your fingertips. Kids love nothing more than to be chased, to be pushed on a swing, to play catch, to simply be active. Your kids can be great role models. If you are playing with your kids, you are killing two birds with one hop, skip, and a jump. Not only are you fostering a loving relationship with your child, but you are also taking care of yourself by being active because, as we saw above, physical activity comes with a plethora of benefits. Bonus: You are teaching your kids lifelong healthy habits.

You can continue to make excuses why you can't, or you can simply make it happen. The human body is incredibly adaptable and is willing to deliver almost anything you ask of it. By just pushing your body beyond what it is currently capable of doing, you will promote the development of strength and endurance. It really is that simple. In fact, the Mayo Clinic suggests that 150 minutes of moderate activity a week is enough to reap all the benefits exercise has to offer. That's only about 20 minutes a day.

You can do anything for twenty minutes!

In fact, that's one of our mantras on The Biggest Loser campus. If you can't do it for twenty minutes to start, you can certainly do it for one minute. Because "you can do anything for one minute." And the next day, you can probably do anything for two minutes. If you only add a minute a day, in just three weeks, you will be able to do anything for twenty minutes.

I've often heard people say, "I'm not like one of those gym people. I just don't enjoy exercise." Don't believe the myth that all those who work out regularly wake up excited to hit the gym or take a jog. That just isn't true. Most people don't have an innate desire to get it done daily and struggle to put in the time and effort. But the reason they continue to exercise regularly is because they have experienced its rewards and want to continue reaping the benefits. So ride your bike to the store, do bodyweight exercises throughout the day, hike the local canyon, stroll around the block, join an online yoga class from your living room, or simply wade through a pool if your knees are barking at you. The world that God placed us in offers endless opportunities to make activity and exercise a part of our daily rituals. All you have to do is delete the words "I can't" from your vocabulary so you can see the possibilities in what you are currently capable of doing. Just move, and you will quickly see the advantages.

"Do not let what you cannot do interfere with what you can do." —John Wooden

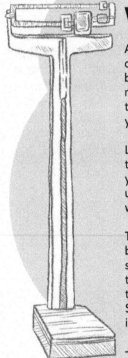

WEIGHING IN

As you start to move your body and eat with a clear conscience, you will begin to see that your body is the best friend you've ever had. It is patient, allows you to make mistakes, never judges you, and is the most loyal thing in your life. All it asks in return? Consistency from you.

Like any relationship, it grows deeper over time through shared experiences. So I encourage you to use your workouts, meals, and moods to help guide your understanding of your body and learn about what's working for you or not!

There's no way to measure this relationship with your body, and certainly a number on a scale will not do, so you must look further than the scale. Because even though weight loss may be a part of your journey, in truth, it is only a side effect of the real wins within you. So remain consistent, and you won't just reach your goals in and out of the gym, you will own them.

—Jen Widerstrom, Bestselling author, fitness director of SHAPE Magazine, and undefeated coach on *The Biggest Loser.*

Episode 2:
NUTRITION

Now that you are moving, you will probably get hungry, so let's move to the kitchen to talk about nutrition. Nutrition is the process of providing the food necessary for health, growth, and repair of the human body. For Megan, like many of us, nutrition was a serious struggle. The means by which she was attempting to fuel her system backfired. She was consuming excessive empty calories that didn't offer her body the nutrients it needed to be healthy, strong, and vibrant.

When you nourish your body properly with the foods that support your system, you'll get a huge return on your investment with all of these benefits:

Proper nutrition...

- Reduces risk of heart disease
- Reduces risk of stroke
- Reduces risk of some cancers
- Lowers your blood pressure
- Controls high cholesterol
- Controls depression and anxiety
- Improves bone and tissue strength
- Increases energy levels
- Aids your immune system in fighting off illness
- Improves recovery time after injury
- Improves the health of your gut
- Improves memory
- Improves sleep
- And, when you are properly nourished, you can control your weight.

Can you see why Hippocrates said, "Our food should be our medicine and our medicine should be our food"?

The dish on eating right

While everyone knows it is important to eat right, not everyone understands what that means. With all of the claims that different diet programs promise, it's understandable that nutrition can be confusing. It would take several degrees in food science to know which one is right. But before you hit the books, you should know that diets tend to go in and out of fashion. Remember the grapefruit and cookie diets of the seventies, the cabbage soup and liquid diets in the eighties, the low fat era of the nineties, and, of course, the Subway diet in 2000? Since then, we have seen apple cider vinegar, baby food, and juice cleanses all vying for our attention and buy-in as a solution to our quest for the perfect food. But here is what you need to know. No one food or diet plan is right for everyone, and by no means are any of them a cure-all solution.

And when we talk solutions, we aren't just talking weight loss. In fact, nutrition is not about weight loss at all. Losing and maintaining a healthy weight just happen to be one of the fringe benefits of eating the foods that nourish and support our body's health. Proper nutrition should be about fueling our bodies so we are capable of navigating the world efficiently and effectively, as well as providing our bodies with the ability to become resilient and restorative. The way to achieve this is through variety, moderation, wholesomeness, and contentment.[vii] (I added in the fourth element contentment, as I have witnessed how being satisfied in life plays a big role in how we choose to feed our bodies.)

Garden variety

A lack of variety in your diet deprives your body of all the nutrients it needs to perform optimally. Choosing a variety of food, instead of thinking that one ingredient or food group is a cure-all, gives your body an opportunity to utilize various nutrients so it can deliver what you require of it daily. They say that "variety is the spice of life," which reminds me to advocate for the many unused spices in your kitchen as well. Spices not only delight the taste buds, but they also offer powerful health benefits. For instance, cinnamon and garlic are beneficial for heart health, while turmeric is known for reducing inflammation in the body and brain. Cayenne, in addition to warming toes when sprinkled in the winter boots of upstate New York kids, is celebrated for easing pain and reducing ulcers. [viii] And that's only the beginning. Give your Lazy Susan a whirl and see what nature has hiding in your spice cabinet.

Moderation in all things, including moderation

We can't all "eat right" all the time, and that's okay. Consuming foods in moderation allows you to supply your body with the nourishment it needs and still treat yourself, now and again, to the delicious foods of this world that aren't necessarily considered "healthy."

A few years after her season aired, a very successful former contestant came to my home for a visit. My husband suggested that we take her to a local milkshake shop on a cliff overlooking the beach. Although one of my favorite places to take out of town visitors, instantly red flags went up in my head knowing the struggles with food she had overcome. She must have sensed my hesitation and said, "Don't worry, I've discovered moderation."

Eating in moderation gives you flexibility and allows you to develop a healthier relationship with food. Instead of eliminating "junk food" all together, moderation provides the freedom to enjoy various cuisine in a more controlled capacity.

The wholesome truth

Wholesomeness refers to choosing foods that are more natural and less processed. When my kids were young and asked for treats in the cookie aisle, I used to say, "I can't buy them because they're too processed." Then one day after school, my son brought home a bag of store-bought cookies, took one bite, and said, "I can taste the process." As a general rule, naturally occurring foods have greater nutritional value than their processed cousins; therefore, they are more beneficial when it comes to supporting and healing your body. An easy way to locate and shop for more wholesome foods is to stick to the perimeter of the store. In most stores, the outer aisles are where you will find fruits, vegetables, meat, fish, and dairy. It's like driving the Indy 500; nothing good comes out of spending your time in the center of the track.

Happy hour

In our fast-paced, stress-charged world, food all too often becomes less about healing and more about coping. We tend to reach for something to put in our mouth every time we are the least bit unsettled. When food is used to subvert whatever ails us, including stress, anger, depression, loneliness, or any of our other emotions, then food is no longer being used as sustenance; it becomes an idol. This is because we are trying to work through our issues with Dolly Madison instead of working through our issues with Jesus Christ. When we seek contentment not in food but in our relationships, especially our relationship with Christ, we find lasting satisfaction and are less subject to the lure of the kitchen pantry.

Food for thought

So how do we fuel and satisfy our bodies and avoid the pitfalls of letting our food control us? If I could boil down (pun intended) this topic and provide you with the two most life-altering upgrades you can make when it comes to proper nutrition, I would tell you to eat at home and control your portion size.

There's no place like home, there's no place like home!

You might be surprised to learn that the contestants on *The Biggest Loser* make all of their own meals while they're on the show. There are no chefs, no boxed meals, and no takeaway delivery, making for an interesting social experiment in the kitchen. We have seen every level of cook, from those who could bring home the bacon but couldn't even identify the frying pan, to others who were so good in the kitchen, they could make the onions cry. And of course every level in between. But regardless of ability, one thing they all had in common was that they all found new ways to produce edible and nutritious food. I can guarantee you, if they can do it in a matter of weeks while competing to lose weight and appearing on national television, you can too! Julia Child reminds us, "The only real stumbling block is fear of failure. In cooking, you've got to have a what-the-hell attitude."

So what the hell, let's look at the reasons cooking at home can benefit you and your loved ones when it comes to nutrition.

⊕ Cooking at home reduces the amount of salt, fat, sugar, artificial flavor, artificial color, and preservatives in your food.

⊕ You choose how your food is cooked and can select nutrient-preserving options (e.g., steaming or grilling vegetables instead of frying them).

⊕ You control the quality of produce, meats, and dairy that you consume.

⊕ Seasonal benefits year round! You can select your own herbs and spices to add flavor that isn't laden with salt and other preservatives.

⊕ You save money. We are talking tons of dough here!

⊕ Because you will feel a sense of pride and accomplishment when you make your own meals, you are more likely to savor every bite, slow down your consumption, and actually enjoy the meal. Cooking is therapy!

⊕ You are acquiring a valuable life skill and will learn heaps about the ingredients that fuel your body. When you increase your knowledge about what you are feeding your body, you will be more discerning with what you put in it. You know what they say, you can't look like a million bucks if you order off the dollar menu!

⊕ Cooking at home is a great way to spend time with your friends and family and get them thinking about their own nutrition. You might be surprised by what you learn about each other while making a big pot of spaghetti sauce or kneading bread together.

Besides, people who can cook are much more interesting!

◉ You can control your portion size (the second most important aspect of nutrition).

Divide and conquer

JJ, a college football player, had always been a big boy. He had struggled with his weight for years but was finally on the road to a lighter and brighter future as a contestant on *The Biggest Loser: Glory Days*. One evening during filming, the cast had to eat at a local takeout joint due to a hectic location shoot. When JJ arrived back at the ranch, I asked him how he had done with his choices at the sandwich shop. JJ got suddenly reflective and said, "I ordered a small drink. In my whole life, I have never ordered anything small. My mom always ordered an extra large or super-size because I was a big kid, and she assumed that's what I needed. Turns out... a small was enough."

When you have paid for and are handed a certain amount of food, chances are you will finish it whether you have had enough or not. But when you eat at home, you can take control of your portion size and only consume what you need.

We had a simple life hack in The Biggest Loser kitchen to help our contestants with portion control: smaller plates.

We are constantly seduced into thinking that bigger is better. We are coaxed into supersizing for a lower price and persuaded to get refills for just a dollar more. They all seem like great deals until that becomes our norm. The next time you are out, give the almost forgotten small a try. You might be surprised that it is actually enough.

> *If you have found honey, eat only enough for you, lest you be sated with it and vomit it.*
> —*Proverbs 25:16*

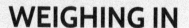

WEIGHING IN

Two words come to mind when asked about nutrition: balance and sustainability. A variety of nutrients are necessary to make sure our bodies have everything they need. That can easily be attained by gracing our plates with a range of colorful fruits and vegetables, proteins, and carbohydrates. Yup, that's right... even carbs are an important part of a balanced diet. Simply remember that life-nurturing changes to the way you eat need to be sustainable for the long haul without feeling restrictive or punishing. By shifting the focus from being a certain size to being healthy, you are choosing a more sustainable path and one that will benefit you throughout your life.

As Remy said in Ratatouille, "This much I know. If you are what you eat, then I only want to eat the good stuff."

—**Katie Chapmon**, *MS, RD. The Biggest Loser Dietitian 2020*

Episode 3:
HYDRATION

My youngest son yelled down from bed one night, "Mom, can you bring me a glass of water?"

I yelled back, "Mick, you are supposed to be asleep. Go to bed!"

About ten minutes later, he yelled down, "Mom, can you bring me a glass of water?"

"Mick, you are supposed to be asleep. If I hear your voice again, you will get a spankin'."

About ten minutes later, he yelled down, "Mom! When you come up to give me a spankin', can you bring me a glass of water?"

It's an old joke… one I have probably used too many times to make this point. As adults, we have forgotten how important water is for our bodies. Do you remember when you were a kid, drinking water straight from the hose on a hot day or sticking your head under the faucet because you were too thirsty to get a glass?

Our bodies crave water because they are made up of water. Our muscles—our ability to work—are about 75 percent water. Our blood—our body's transportation system—is 50 percent water. And our brain—our capacity to think, process, and react—is approximately 80–85 percent water. [ix] In the Bible, water is often used symbolically to represent cleansing, healing, and life. But truthfully, it shouldn't be a symbol at all because water in fact does cleanse, heal, and give us life. Our body needs water not only to survive but also to thrive.

When you are properly hydrated, by drinking a sufficient amount of water daily, you will find:

- Your muscles and joints work better. It's like lubrication in a car.
- Your back pain will diminish.

⊕ You will speed recovery. Your body heals faster when it has all the right elements.

⊕ You'll have a healthier heart.

⊕ You will be able to control your cholesterol levels.

⊕ You will cleanse toxins from your body. It's like giving our insides a bath.

⊕ You will help eliminate digestive disorders. Literally flush them away!

⊕ Your organ function improves.

⊕ You'll sleep better and fight dreaded afternoon fatigue because dehydration, or lack of water, is the number one cause of daytime drowsiness.

And if all that isn't enough, another huge bonus is hydration helps you keep your skin soft and supple and actually slows the aging process. As it turns out, the fountain of youth is literally the water fountain!

Soda-pressing

Sugary drinks are the largest source of calories and added sugar in the US diet.[x] We have replaced that desperate need for water with much lesser fluids that are often nothing more than chemicals, artificial flavors, and colors. Unfortunately for our bodies, these sugar-laden fluids do not support our systems, and therefore, our bodies do not work as efficiently and effectively as they should and could if we simply fueled them with what they desire and deserve.

In The Biggest Loser house, as you can imagine, the majority of our contestants arrive addicted to soft drinks, but not for long. Soda is one of the first sugar-charged drinks to be removed from our contestants' diets. Although sugar is highly addictive, when our contestants weren't able to access a sweet, carbonated beverage to satisfy their cravings, we discovered it wasn't necessarily the sweetness they craved, but the effervescence of the drink. This was quickly remedied with easy-to-use kitchen counter carbonation machines. The contestants flavored their new bubbly waters by combining fresh fruit, herbs, and honey to create healthy syrups that were "sodalicious." They were happy to leave their old habit behind. So if you are looking to cut back or preferably eliminate your soft drink intake, "get busy with the fizzy" as Soda Stream encourages, and see what healthy, natural, and mouthwatering beverages you can create.

Water you waiting for?

You know what we say in the hydration business: "More water in your gut will keep you off of your butt!" Try to remember that hydration is an ongoing process. Managing your water intake throughout the day is important for the health of your whole body. However, don't beat yourself up with water math, trying to figure out the exact number of ounces you require in a twenty-four hour period. Some days are more challenging than others. The key is to listen to your body and make choices that support your anatomy instead of choices that undermine all of the other work you are putting into living a healthy life. To get the right fluid into your system daily, try these easy-to-implement strategies:

- Drink a glass of water with every meal, and pause to take a swig of water before snacking. You might discover by snackciddent that you aren't even hungry; you were just thirsty!
- Fill your water container at the beginning of the day, and don't go to bed before it's finished. You'll want to drink it throughout the day so the last chug isn't keeping you up at night.
- My personal favorite intake approach is to chew your fluids. This is easy with high-water-content food like watermelon, cantaloupe, cucumbers, strawberries, oranges, and lettuce, to name a few.
- See the "Weighing In" section at the end of this chapter for some additional pro tips from a hydration specialist!

Remember, if you're thirsty, that's your body's warning system telling you it's time to refill what you've lost. So go ahead, stick your head under the faucet, and remember how great it feels to give your body not only what it needs to survive but also to thrive.

> *He is like a tree planted by streams of water, that yields its fruit in its season, and its leaf does not wither. In all that he does, he prospers.*
> *—Psalm 1:3*

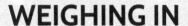

WEIGHING IN

Staying hydrated is not as hard as it sounds, but also not as easy as it sounds. A great rule of thumb to know where your hydration levels stand is checking the color of your urine: the clearer, the better! Think of your body as a machine, and water as the oil. Our bodies need water to function smoothly and for long periods of time, just like a machine needs oil. But having too much or too little can be hazardous. Some of my favorite tips to share with people who need help drinking more water are so simple!

Tip #1: Always carry a water bottle (preferably a reusable one). It helps to have a visual reminder and/or cue to drink more often.

Tip #2: Try using a straw. Some people (myself included) find it helps you drink water faster without even noticing it.

Tip #3: Make it taste good! Don't like the taste of water? Add lemon, cucumbers, oranges, or a flavored (sugarless) additive.

"If there is magic on this planet, it is contained in water."
— Loren Eiseley (American anthropologist)

—**Smadar Bezalel**, *MS, ATC, CSCS, CES, PES, former athletic trainer on The Biggest Loser*

Episode 4:
RECOVERY

A good laugh and a long sleep are the two best cures for anything.
—Irish proverb

Now that you have been moving, eating right, and staying hydrated, I would imagine that you are exhausted. That's perfect because our next step is to get you some proper recovery time or, simply, sleep!

Sleep is incredibly important for the upkeep of our bodies. The human body, like most incredible machines, can only go so long with little to no care. Rest is the daily maintenance plan you need to avoid premature breakdown. So often we deny our body the recovery time it requires to heal and then force it to keep up the next day, loading it up with chemicals and supplements to keep it running at any cost. And it is usually those chemicals and supplements that interfere with our sleep the next night. It's a vicious cycle that needs to be broken because successful sleep is truly the only way to make our bodies work efficiently and effectively and to extend the life of these extraordinary machines.

When you have given your body the gift of sleep, you will:

- Experience less stress and anxiety
- Reduce depression
- Give your body time to repair and heal itself
- Reduce inflammation
- Regulate blood sugar
- Reduce blood pressure
- Increase your immunity

⊕ Keep your heart healthy
⊕ Improve brain function
⊕ Lose more weight

And get this: when you get proper rest, you can actually improve your romantic life. And we all thought we needed to be awake in bed to improve our romantic life! Turns out, lack of sleep can directly affect our relationships by interfering with and often obstructing our emotions.[xi] When we can't manage our feelings or regulate our reactions, our relationships are sure to suffer. This is especially true of our passionately charged relationships. You know the old saying "never go to bed angry." Well, it's just that, an old saying. I would suggest that you call a timeout, get a good night's sleep, and continue where you left off in the morning. Likely, you will both be more levelheaded when you approach the discussion the next day, and equitable discussions during the day make for better connections under the sheets at night.

> *There was never a night or a problem that could defeat sunrise or hope.*
> —*Bernard Williams (English moral philosopher)*

Slumber party

The rules haven't changed. According to the Center for Disease Control, adults need seven or more hours and teens need eight–ten hours of sleep per night in order for their bodies to fully recover and heal from the demands put on them daily.[xii] If you haven't had your head on a pillow for the exact number of hours nightly, don't lose sleep over it. Simply start a habit of recovery that will provide your body all it needs to flourish in our challenging world. The next time you turn in, implement these tried-and-true strategies that have helped lull our contestants to sleep so they too could catch up on some much-needed z's.

Heavy blankets are a miracle for those who suffer from restless sleep.

Blankets with additional weight sewn into them help reduce tossing and turning and allow the user a more restful slumber. Think of it like swaddling a baby. When my kids were little, I made weighted blankets that were ten percent of their body weight but soon discovered how beneficial they were for adults, and in no time, I was crafting twenty-pound blankets on the regular. I've made so many weighted blankets I can sew them in my sleep! Thank goodness you can purchase them just about anywhere today!

By rewinding your day, you can put to bed the idea that you can't fall asleep. Backwards day is a simple visualization exercise to slow down and reverse your thought cycle. In this exercise, you simply recount the events of your day; however, this time you imagine them backward or in reverse order. Within a couple of minutes, your brain will stop charging forward, you will slow down your thinking, begin to relax, and will soon be out like a light.

Lastly, I wouldn't dream of putting this subject to rest, without letting you know that the best way to get better sleep is through the other three components of physical health: exercise, proper nutrition, and hydration. Each of the body essentials, when done right, increases your quality of sleep, and sleep improves the overall health of your body. One contestant showed how much the other elements improved his sleep and, in turn, his life, in my favorite non-scale win. Non-scale wins are the victories that our contestants experience while on their weight-loss journey that have nothing to do with the scale. They are the everyday indicators that reflect a healthier lifestyle. This can be fitting into an old pair of jeans, not needing a seat belt extender on a plane, getting up off the floor without help, decreasing medication, or in this case eliminating snoring.

When Jim arrived home after being on The Biggest Loser campus for over three months, he reported that it was the first time in years that he and his wife were able to go to bed together. Due to Jim's weight, he suffered from sleep apnea, a serious sleep disorder in which breathing repeatedly stops and starts throughout the night. One of the symptoms of sleep apnea is chronic, loud snoring. Because of his excessive snoring, his wife had a difficult time falling asleep each night, so she would head to bed hours before Jim began to "saw logs." You know what they say: "Laugh, and the world laughs with you; snore, and you sleep alone."[xiii] When Jim started to exercise, eat right, and drink more water, his sleep apnea disappeared along with his snoring, and not only was he able to get a good night sleep for the first time in years but he was also able to enjoy the company of his wife, who, by the way, was finally getting a good night sleep as well.

Give yourself the gift of recovery, and your body will surprise you. You might be capable of so much more than you ever imagined.

The disciples said to him, "Lord, if he has fallen asleep, he will recover." —John 11:12

WEIGHING IN

Sleep is the number one recovery tool you have at your disposal, and second place isn't even close. If you aren't getting enough, there is nothing else you can do to make it up. No expensive machine, new technology, or app can help a lack of sleep. Sleep deprivation can leave you more susceptible to injury and illness, not to mention the way it makes you feel. Sleep is the time when your body is able to repair any damage, good or bad, that you do to it during the day. You can rebuild muscle and repair tissue. Your body can reset and recharge. In short, sleep should be your main priority when it comes to recovery.

As Benjamin Franklin said, "Early to bed and early to rise makes a man healthy, wealthy, and wise."

—**Carlos Olivas**, *LAT, ATC. Athletic trainer for the Nashville Sound AAA baseball team and athletic trainer on The Biggest Loser 2020*

Season Finale:

BODY

So we have just discussed the quadfecta of physical health. Now the cool thing about these four components is that they work with and for each other. I already mentioned how the first three improve your sleep, but let me explain further. When you start to exercise, you will inevitably be thirsty. When you drink more water to quench that thirst, you will cleanse the toxins from your body, and you will crave healthier foods. When you feed your body the right nutrients and hydrate it properly, you will sleep better. When you sleep better, you will have more energy to exercise.

So that, my friends, is why we always start our contestants in the gym because when you affect one area of your physical health, the others will simply fall into place. But no matter where you start, each component of physical health will lead you to the others.

When Megan started a regular routine of exercise, she quickly realized that she needed to get her nutrition and hydration in check in order to fuel her body for the demands she was placing on it. Healthier habits emerged, and she happily left behind the things that weren't supporting her new lifestyle and allowing her to advance toward wellness.

Megan went on to win *The Biggest Loser* at-home prize for maintaining weight-loss following elimination from the show. She continues to make healthy choices that will inevitably heal her body and says that the tools she learned to lose weight have transferred to all areas of her life. Her biggest takeaway is that you have to be willing to ask for help. Having the courage to ask for and accept help on her journey of healing gave Megan the power to lose what wasn't serving her and gain a new lease on life. Megan's success reminds me that by doing the basics and doing them well, you can easily move in the direction of wellness. Follow her on Instagram @iamhoffy to see where her transformation takes her next.

When my favorite author, Matthew Kelly, wrote this, he might not have been talking about physical health, but I do believe his words are incredibly appropriate here:

Success at almost anything rests upon this single principle: Do the basics, do them well, and do them every day, especially when you don't feel like doing them.

I have just given you the body basics. They are the keys to successfully healing your body. And remember, it's not about where you start, it's the fact that you simply start that makes all the difference in this healing journey.

Where will your journey begin?

Season 3

MIND

Scott's Story

"Do not be conformed to this world but be transformed by the renewal of your mind, that you may prove what is the will of God, what is good and acceptable and perfect."
—Roman 12:2

Scott, a six-foot-six-inch, 366-pound former NFL quarterback, had recently lost his father after a long and intense battle with type 2 diabetes. While Scott struggled in numerous areas of his life, it was evident he had dropped the ball when it came to maintaining his weight. That's when he decided to audition for *The Biggest Loser: Glory Days*. This particular season featured former athletes that had been sidelined by their weight.

Clearly an elite athlete, Scott should have been able to bring his A game when it came to his physique. So how did he end up on a weight loss show? Well, for the first couple of weeks on the ranch, he played Monday morning quarterback trying to figure out exactly how he landed at this place in his life. What he discovered about himself was that, in addition to his physical struggle, he was also fighting an emotional battle after losing his father to an obesity-related disease. On some level, Scott recognized that because of his weight gain, he was likely headed for the same fate. But instead of facing that realization head-on and doing something about it, he packed on the pounds both physically and emotionally—carrying with him fear, humiliation, pain, and of course immense sadness for the loss of his father. Mental baggage for most is much harder to carry than physical baggage, but both will keep you from living your best life.

It wasn't too late in the game for Scott to tackle his weight issues and break the cycle of obesity in his family. But in order to do so, he would first have to create a game plan to cultivate a healthy mind. No surprise, his plan revolved around an offensive attack.

Any quarterback that understands what the offense is really about is going to succeed.
—*Joe Montana*

Scott implemented strategies to further understand and process his thoughts, feelings, and emotions, and when he did this, it hit him like a lineman on a blitz. He finally realized that his mental game was directly affecting his overall state of health. So he took essential strides to heal the wounds of his mind as well as his body. It was a quarterback sneak that took him right into the end zone. One day, he was just an overweight guy on a treadmill trying to survive the workout, and the next he was an NFL quarterback leading his team to victory. It was one of the most amazing transformations I have ever seen, and it happened when he told his mind to get out of his body's way. Sound advice from his trainer!

The approach that Scott used didn't come out of a playbook, but nonetheless was a game-changer in helping him reshape his thought process and heal his mind, and as a result, his body. I hope these seven strategies kick off a new way of thinking so that you too can experience days of glory and wellness.

"Are you ready for some ~~foot~~ *MIND*ball?"

Episode 5:
DETERMINE YOUR WHY

Aside from always having front-row seats, one of the best things about being an athletic trainer is the potential to hear an exceptional coach's halftime talk. I've always liked the idea that you could take a group of people who were on the verge of giving up, and with your words, if they were strung together with power, eloquence, and a touch of hope, you could lead the defeated to victory.

When I started practicing sports medicine outside of sports, I genuinely missed those awe-inspiring twelve-minute football locker room pep talks that often made the difference between winning and losing. I decided long ago to make "halftime talks" a part of my repertoire, no matter what population I am working with. So before our contestants set off on a challenge or step into the gym for the first time, I gather them up and do my very best to thread together words that embolden and inspire so they too come out on the other side victorious.

Why? What's the big deal?

"Determine your why" has become one of my most exercised halftime talks because truly knowing the reason that you are doing something, especially when that something is challenging, demanding, or just downright scary, will make all the difference in deciding whether to quit or carry on. And in life, that decision dictates whether you win or lose. So in case you are facing a formidable opponent in your life, these inspirational words strung together with a message of hope about discovering and using your why will help you confront any opposition:

German philosopher Nietzsche said, "He who has a WHY can endure any how."

So, I want you to think for a second... why are you here? Why are you on this voyage? Who or what is motivating you to live a better life at this point in time?

At this very moment, determining your why will drastically change the outcome of this journey. Your why will motivate you when you want to quit, it will drive you forward, it will keep you focused, and most importantly, your why will give you the courage to take the first step. And sometimes the smallest step in the right direction ends up being the biggest step of your life.

Scott's why was his desire to break the cycle of obesity in his family so he and his children could live long, healthy lives. When the workouts were taking a toll on his body, and quitting seemed easier than enduring another week away from his loved ones, it was his why that fueled his desire to persevere and continue striving for his ultimate goal. Sonya, former contestant and collegiate All-American softball player said, "Your why will remind you that your personal convictions are greater than your present circumstances." And although one of Scott's biggest competitors that season, I believe he would agree with her on that!

Why not now?

A simple way to establish your why is to make a list of your priorities and rank them from highest to lowest. That way, everything you do and every decision you make can be weighed against the list. For instance, if your top priority is spending time with your family, you can comfortably make a decision when offered the opportunity to pick up an additional shift at work over the weekend. Your why permits you to say no because it doesn't support your top priority of spending time with your family. However, if advancing your career or making extra money for the holidays ranked number one on your list, then your why encourages you to take on the extra hours and benefit from the additional work. Neither is better than the other; it's just a matter of priority. Likewise, if living a healthy life registers high on your list, then taking the steps necessary to facilitate that lifestyle will be a piece of cake, or something healthier than cake! Just remember that your list will change as you change, and your priorities will be different when you are different. The list is fluid and needs to be updated often; that way, you can make sure that your priorities are in order and easily determine your why.

So before you do anything else, even before you read another chapter, figure out your why. Why are you reading this book? Are you looking to heal a specific part of your life? Do you want to shed an old habit that's holding you back? Is there more in this world that you want to experience? Is God calling you to something bigger and better? Find your answer and then use that reason to take the next step, because every step you take forward leads you closer to victory.

WEIGHING IN

When I set out to write this book, I had forgotten why I was doing it and often found myself distracted from the project. And when I wasn't distracted, I was doubtful that I had something worth writing. My why reminded me that there is power and purpose in the written word and that if one person is led to healing and ultimately wellness through my book, it was worth every tap of the keyboard. My why is you, the person reading this book. You are the reason I kept writing. And it is through writing this book that I healed as well. So I owe you a great deal of thanks. After reading Simon Sinek's book Start with Why: How Great Leaders Inspire Everyone to Take Action, I remember to apply a why to everything in my life. If you are still not convinced of the power of why, or you just want to hear more about how this three-letter word can make or break just about anything you set out to do, then give his book a read. You'll stop asking why and start using it to lead you forward.

—Kelly

Episode 6:

PARTICIPATE IN SUPPORT GROUPS

You can find numerous ways to make connections with people who will support your efforts to grow and change for the better. One good way is competing for $250,000 on a reality TV show. But don't worry if you haven't been cast on a popular weight-loss program where you'll struggle through your most personal moments before millions of viewers around the world. You can still find fellowship, unity, and service that will benefit you and everyone you have a relationship with through a support group.

Support groups work for a reason. When members of a group can share similar experiences and freely express fear, anxiety, resentments, and disappointments, as well as celebrate personal victories and triumphs, each of the members discover that the issues they're facing are not theirs alone to solve.

Support groups allow us to look at ourselves with greater clarity through a stranger's story that resonates with our own. We soon realize that we share the same challenges as others in our community, revealing that we are not alone. Laughing, crying, and openly talking with others in similar situations allows us to create intimate bonds of trust and acceptance. In turn, these bonds allow us to be vulnerable so we can fully express our thoughts and feelings. And when we do that, we can address things about ourselves and our situation that would have otherwise been too difficult to face.

I listened to their stories and found so many areas where we overlapped—not all the deeds, but the feelings of remorse and hopelessness.
—The Big Book of Alcoholics Anonymous

Scott, familiar with the idea of teammates from his years of playing football, easily created these necessary supportive bonds with his fellow cast members, as do the majority of the contestants on the show. Although they are initially competing for a grand prize, they always discover a camaraderie in working toward a common goal. These bonds inevitably develop into deep friendships. Not surprising! Together they can laugh, share personal stories, express anger, and cry—all without judgement. But most importantly, they can encourage each other and provide understanding and acceptance when they need it most. Support groups empower individuals to face their demons and rise above them.

But not everyone is excited about the idea of joining a support group. I get it! There is something very real and very scary about sharing your struggles with someone else, especially strangers. To these folks, I offer the same words I reiterate to our contestants over and over again throughout the filming season:

"Trust the process!"

There are people who have come before you and figured it out so you don't have to. Don't be afraid to seek and ask for support. People want to share what they have lived and learned.

"Trust the process!"

The most successful peer support organizations in the world rely on the fundamental principles of fellowship, unity, and service.

"Trust the process!"

When you have a safe place to be vulnerable with people who understand what you are going through and can express empathy for your situation, you will begin to heal.

"Trust the process!"

Support groups create a network of individuals that can look past themselves and their own issues in service of others. And when you serve others, you will naturally heal yourself and edge closer to wellness.

"Trust the process!"

> *The future is, most of all, in the hands of those people who recognize the other as a "you" and themselves as part of an "us." We all need each other.*
> —*Pope Francis*

Two's company, three's a support group

There are numerous ways to locate groups that can support you through life's toughest challenges. Your primary care physician or mental health professional may have access to reputable groups in your area, but if not, uncovering one that fits your needs is as easy as an internet search. Some great national resources for finding the group that's right for you are:

- Psychology Today: https://www.psychologytoday.com/us/groups

- NAMI: National Alliance on Mental Illness: https://www.nami. org/Support-Education

- Support Groups Central: https://www.supportgroupscentral.com/index.cfm

And here is a wonderfully detailed article that can help you find the support group that meets your specific needs: How Can I Find A Support Group Meeting Near Me. https://www.verywellmind.com/find-a-support-group-meeting-near-you-69433

In case you haven't found the right group just yet but still need support, you can always reach an empathetic ear and a reassuring voice on a crisis text line. In the US and Canada, simply text 741741 (85258/UK and 50808/Ireland) or visit their site at https://www.crisistextline.org to connect with a crisis counselor.

Remember, support groups don't always have to be formal. If you can find a common bond within your circle of friends, family, small faith group, or volunteer organization, then by all means lean into the people who already love you and are willing to support you through any of the challenges you face in life.

WEIGHING IN

Groups and support groups have an amazing capacity for healing and self-understanding. They have the power to help you feel understood by others who have gone through similar experiences so you don't feel alone on the journey. They can also provide the magic ingredient of instilling hope. Hope is what keeps us going in life and can ultimately heal us—the hope that it is possible to change, to live a more fulfilling life, to take better care of ourselves, our health, our hearts, our souls, and each other. Groups can give us the fuel we need to become a role model for the kind of life we want to live, experience, and share with the world

—Patricia A. Velazquez, *PhD, Psychotherapist for The Biggest Loser 2020.*

Episode 7:
BECOME AND STAY ACTIVE

To keep the body in good health is a duty, otherwise we shall not be able to keep our mind strong and clear.
– Buddha

Ten years after being on *The Biggest Loser*, Brittany, a former contestant, found herself in one of the darkest places of her life. She was the heaviest she had ever been and was learning to navigate grief and depression after the sudden passing of her mother. She realized that no one was coming to rescue her from this dark place, so she consciously made a choice to rewrite her story. In a moment of clarity, she decided to sell the last gift her mother gave her to purchase a Peloton stationary bike for her home. It has been a few years now, and Brittany has maintained her healthy weight and continues to ride almost daily. I have been on Zoom calls with Brittany where she's literally along for the ride, as she pedals away on her chrome pony throughout the meeting. The bike offers a wonderful program for her physical health, but reprogramming her mind to show up for herself even when she had every excuse not to is why she is able to sit tall in her saddle today.

To aid in healing their mind, our contestants must stay active. Turns out, that's not too hard to do on a nationally televised weight-loss show! But physical activity proves to be more rewarding than simply a component of healing the body. It also plays a huge role in healing and developing a healthy mind.

When we are active, we increase blood flow to the brain, and without getting too "sciencey," we create chemical reactions that benefit how we think and how we feel.

Physical activity can protect against cognitive decline and stave off anxiety and depression. According to the Mayo Clinic, exercising for thirty minutes or more a day, three to five days a week will significantly reduce symptoms of depression and anxiety.[xiv] Even as little as ten to fifteen minutes at a time can make a considerable impact when it comes to mental health. Hundreds of studies prove how physical activity can relieve and often eliminate stress, anxiety, and depression. I have seen it countless times myself.

When our contestants arrive on campus, they inevitably have a bag full of pills and potions. Some of it's over the counter, and some of it's prescription. But a great deal of their medication is to aid in the reduction of anxiety and depression-related conditions. The majority of contestants who arrive with substances to control symptoms of anxiety and depression are freed from them as soon as they start a consistent routine of physical activity. They simply no longer need the medication. If you remember back to our list of the benefits of exercise, you will be in a better mood because physical activity fights depression and reduces stress and anxiety! (Please remember that our contestants are medically supervised. People do have conditions or chemical imbalances that require the use of specific drugs, so always seek medical advice prior to reducing, eliminating, or altering any medication.)

> *A vigorous five-mile walk will do more good for an unhappy but otherwise healthy adult than all the medicine and psychology in the world.*
> —*Paul Dudley White,* an American physician and cardiologist widely regarded as the founder of preventive cardiology.

Dynamic duo

An older friend of mine once told me that his constant companion, Daisy, was a five-decade dog. I wasn't sure what that meant, so I pressed a little further for clarification. He explained that while his wife was suffering from dementia, she desperately wanted a fuzzy, white lap dog, the kind she saw Betty White holding in a popular commercial that aired during her favorite program. After much hesitation, he finally broke down, and for her birthday, he found her an eleven-pound snow-colored pup, and his wife Donna and sweet Daisy became fast friends. However, he soon realized that in addition to caring for his ailing wife, he would also be the one managing the needs of the dog. One day while walking Daisy, and out of pure boredom he admits, he discovered that the amount of time the dog needed to do her business and return home was the exact amount of time it took him to recite five decades of the rosary. So daily, he and Daisy set out on their excursions, a twenty-minute rosary walk, that they have continued well beyond his wife's passing. I have no doubt that the routine of physical activity that my friend and Daisy shared aided in the healing of his mind as he dealt with the debilitating illness that was robbing his wife of her faculties and eventually her life, and that the rosary and the dog ultimately healed his broken heart.

Remember, physical activity has the power to reduce and eliminate mental stressors. When you alleviate stress, anxiety, and depression, your mind will begin to heal, and you will be one step closer to living your best life and being well. So think about what it is you like doing, set some goals, and start a habit of daily activity. Before you know it, being active and staying active will simply become second nature.

Our lives change when our habits change.
—*Matthew Kelly*

WEIGHING IN

Physical activity reminds me of the divine wisdom in the simple phrase *"put on your own oxygen mask first."*

One of my greatest passions is to take care of other people... to simply meet the needs of others. I love to take care of my friends, my family, my pets, and anyone else that God might put in my path.

What I have learned since *The Biggest Loser* is that if I don't take care of myself the way I should, I simply cannot take care of others the way I want. I've recognized that without physical activity, I don't have the strength or the stamina to take care of those in need. I had to learn to administer oxygen to myself first.

Staying active puts me in a better space physically but also, and most importantly, puts me in a better headspace. I am able to attack the day clear headed, with confidence and boldness, being the best I can be. That way, I can encourage others to be their best selves as well. That's really what it's all about... taking care of me so that I can take care of you. And after all, isn't that His plan. So go ahead and strap on your O2 mask, take a deep breath, and let's all do our part in taking care of each other.

—**Sonya Jones**, *former Biggest Loser finalist, author, motivational speaker, owner of Losin' It with Sonya Jones.*

Episode 8:
PRACTICE MINDFULNESS

For as he thinks within himself, so he is.
—Proverbs 23:7 (NIV)

Rob was one of the most fascinating contestants I had the pleasure of knowing. He was a twenty-six-year-old six-foot-seven-inch 483-pound giant on screen, but off-camera, he was gentle and kind and one of my favorite people to be around. One day, when we were filming in front of the gym, Rob was exhausted from running hills, so he plopped down on the ground to catch his breath. Just then, a brilliant green tree frog jumped into his lap. With such innocence and childlike delight, he started screeching, "Get a camera over here, get a camera... there's a tree frog on my lap." That's when one of the cameramen leaned over to me and said, "Does he know this show's not about tree frogs?" While it may not have been about tree frogs, it was certainly about gaining wellness, and in that moment, Rob was being mindful of his current surroundings and enjoying them, improving his mental health.

Rob had spent most of his life drowning his feelings with food. If a guy that big gets mad, it can be legitimately scary. So instead of expressing his feelings, frustrations, and fears, he would simply eat them away. But what do you think happens to a young man that has never learned how to express or deal with his emotions when you suddenly take away his coping mechanism?

That's right... fireworks, and if you happen to have seen *The Biggest Loser: Glory Days*, you might remember a few of those uncomfortable blowups on camera. What you didn't see was how embarrassed and remorseful Rob was following each of his very public outbursts. He had simply never allowed himself to experience these raw, authentic emotions. So at the time, he was incapable of identifying or processing them. Everything just came out in concentrated rage. And being out of control does not serve our mental well-being.

Mastering our emotions and being in control starts with the practice of mindfulness. According to the Merriam-Webster Dictionary, the definition of mindfulness is "the practice of maintaining a nonjudgmental state of heightened or complete awareness of one's thoughts, emotions, or experiences on a moment-to-moment basis." [xv]

When you pay attention to what you are observing and experiencing, you will encounter a deeper understanding of what you are feeling, and in turn, you will be more capable of controlling your actions. Mindfulness is the ability to be fully present, aware of your thoughts and emotions, of where you are, and what we are doing. The capacity to be fully present allows us to respond appropriately and not overreact or become overwhelmed by what's going on around us.

Do you mind?

Practicing mindfulness means becoming more aware of your thoughts, feelings, and emotions. What we carry around in our head matters. So being aware of the thoughts and emotions that serve us and discarding those that don't is crucial to our mental well-being. If we carry joy, we will become joyful, but if we are carrying around anger, we will inescapably become angry. When we can determine and control our own behaviors, we will naturally feel better about ourselves and our experiences. And when you feel better about yourself and your life experiences, you are consequently enhancing your mental health.

As Buddha said, "Our life is shaped by our minds. We become what we think." So to appropriately shape our minds and become what we want to become, just like anything else, we must first practice. Here are three mindfulness practices that can easily be embraced and made a part of your daily routine.

Chew on this

We all eat, right? But do we do it mindfully? Meals provide three opportunities a day to practice mindfulness because focusing your attention on the meal in front of you, how it looks, smells, and tastes; where it came from; and the effort it took to make it to your table allows you to feel more satisfied and nourished after consuming it.

When my kids were little, I realized that I was spending hours in the kitchen preparing dinner each day only to have everyone wolf it down, scatter from the table, and head back to their rooms. The whole experience was over in a matter of minutes. So we invented (I use that word loosely) a game we called "Good/Bad." In this game, we each took turns telling those at the table something bad that had happened in our day, and then on the second round, something good that had happened in our day. This became a nightly practice. Here we would listen to each other's successes and failures, offer advice and encouragement, and mostly laugh about the crazy things that happen to each of us daily. It was a source of much conversation.

This simple silly game that we played daily gave us the space to be mindful as we ate. We learned how to express ourselves without fear of ridicule and support one another in our highs and lows. We learned how to listen and be listened to and how to ask questions that encouraged participation. We became mindful of what was at the table before us, including each other. On a side note, our kids, now teenagers and young adults, still want to play, especially when their friends come to dinner.

If you are multitasking, driving, watching TV, working on the computer as you consume your food, or if you are simply racing to get back to what you were doing before your meal, you are missing the emotions and feelings that go along with the experience of eating. You might feel overwhelming gratitude for the farmers who grew and harvested the vegetables on your plate, you might be excited about a new recipe you are trying out for the picky eater in your family, or you could be exasperated that the picky eater won't eat the farm-grown vegetables! But if you're multitasking while eating, those emotions will simply get pushed aside for the other things that you are trying to squeeze into that space.

Mealtime is a great time to be aware of your feelings during the day and in the moment. You will always be more satisfied after a meal where gratitude was experienced, simply because you allowed yourself to be mindful of the feeling.

> So, whether you eat or drink, or whatever you do, do all
> to the glory of God.
> —1 Corinthians 10:31

Change of pace

Nature offers endless opportunities to practice mindfulness. Paying attention to our surroundings, especially the beauty of God's creation, helps us to be more in tune with our own feelings. When we take time to stop and smell the roses, or the cow pasture for that matter, we experience them at a deeper level as more of our senses become involved. When more of our senses are involved, we can be present in the moment and are truly mindful of our intentions and actions.

When I was working in Croatia this past year, on another television show, I couldn't wait to get outside each day because there I saw colors that I didn't know existed outside of a Crayola box. The blues were the most awe-inspiring hues I had ever experienced. That's right—I didn't just see them; I experienced them.

I once heard that if you are helplessly drawn to the blue in the sky, it is Mary reaching out to you, trying to hold your attention. (I really like the idea of this, so I have chosen to believe it as fact!) While taking in the bountiful shades of blue that dominated the sky and the sea, I could actually feel Mary wrapping her mantle around my body and drawing me closer. This allowed me to surrender my many worries to her Son so I could live in the moment that God had created for us. This is nature creating mindfulness.

Both King Gillette Ranch, where *The Biggest Loser* was filmed in previous seasons, and our location outside of Santa Fe, New Mexico, have offered our contestants some of the most beautiful terrains to stroll, hike, jog, and wander in the wonder of God's immense and teeny-tiny creations. In the silence and beauty of nature is where they truly begin to practice mindfulness.

A prayer walk is a great way to be mindful. In case you don't know where to start, just throw on your sneakers and pop in your headphones because there are numerous resources online that offer prayer walks tailored to your specific time constraints. You can even map a prayer route! These resources will guide you and keep you in the moment so that you can focus on the beauty that surrounds you.

> On the glorious splendor of thy majesty, and on thy wondrous works, I will meditate.
> —Psalm 145:5

Take a breather

When expectations are high, cameras are in your face, the workout has drained you physically and mentally, a weigh-in is right around the corner, and your teammates have put their hope in you lasting another three minutes on the treadmill, what is the last thing you are thinking about? Probably breathing! In fact, most of us forget that we can actually control our breathing. Why would you need or even want to control something that's automatic? In the middle of all this pressure, physical stress, and anxiety, shouldn't it be one less thing you have to worry about?

When you are stressed, anxious, or fearful, as our contestants often are, your breathing becomes faster and more shallow, your heart rate speeds up, and your blood pressure increases. In addition, when this happens, you reduce the amount of oxygen you are taking in to fuel your muscles and your brain, so you will inevitably experience both a physical and cognitive decline.

Katarina, a young nurse and recent contestant, would become so anxious during workouts that she would often begin to hyperventilate. She had never pushed herself to physical extremes, and she had a hard time wrapping her brain around the idea that she was capable. So she would become overwhelmingly stressed, anxious, and fearful. And when this happened, she would simply forget to breathe. We must have told her a thousand times, "Kat, just breathe!" With enough encouragement and support to manage her breath through these troubling episodes, she would discover that controlled breathing has incredible power over your body and your mind.

Concentrating on slow, deep breathing helps reduce your heart rate and lower your blood pressure. Your deep inhales are fueling your muscles with oxygen, and your extended exhales transport all of that carbon dioxide waste out of your system. This slow and controlled breathing triggers the parasympathetic nervous system and allows you to feel relaxed and in control. In addition, when you are concentrating on breathing, you are not thinking about the things that are stressing you out and making you anxious. This control is a big piece of being mindful. So set out to do even the most automatic process with purpose, instead of letting your perceptions and emotions trigger physical reactions that are detrimental to your health and well-being.

Did you know that with every breath you take you are speaking the name of God? The word YHWH, or as we pronounce Yahweh (interestingly, a form of God's name that was thought too sacred to be spoken aloud), represents the sound of our very breath. Try it now. Take a deep inhale through your mouth and you will hear the sound "yah." Slowly let it out and you will hear the sound "weh." Once you hear it, you will never un-hear it, and isn't that a gift. Think about this: with our very first breath, we spoke the name of the Lord and, poetically, it will be the last word to pass over our lips as we leave this world. Genius! When I am distracted or overwhelmed, I often employ the practice of slowly and intentionally breathing God's name, Yahweh, Yah-weh, to center my mind and bring me back to Him, where He is always waiting patiently to offer me solace and peace of mind.

> *Let everything that breathes praise the Lord! Praise the Lord!*
> *—Psalm 150:6*

WEIGHING IN

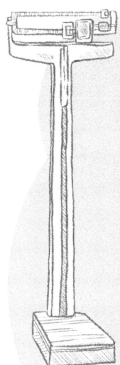

Mindfulness has become a huge part of my life after my experience on *The Biggest Loser*. Learning how mindset can create an environment of perceived "success" or "failure," each year, each day, each moment has been life changing. (I put these words in quotes because all of our experiences can be shifted into either category depending on how we perceive them.)

This chapter reminds me of a song I performed and released while on *The Biggest Loser*. I wrote "Out of the Darkness" many years before when I was in a dark place. I felt like a failure after being a contestant on *The Voice*, but I knew I wanted to change the narrative. Change my perspective.

When we filmed the music video, the crew walked around NYC on a freezing morning carrying a huge (and heavy) mirror. The concept was to strike up conversations with people passing by about how they perceived themselves when they looked in the mirror and how "carrying that weight" of their mirror image daily affected their lives. Not only did we meet some amazing people, but we also had deep conversations with strangers about the impact their mind's eye had on their relationships, their jobs, and their daily choices.

My song "Out of the Darkness" reminds me how powerful a positive (or negative for that matter) mindset can impact outcomes.

"I'll only have myself to blame
If I don't fight to win,
Overcome,
Realize that I'm the only one
Who can save me
Don't let myself get in the way"

—**Erin Willett**, *Semifinalist Season 2 The Voice and The Biggest Loser, Season 17, Contestant*

Episode 9:
LAUGH OUT LOUD

While strolling along the beach, two Biggest Loser contestants, who were sweating excessively through their blue jeans and triple XL T-shirts, noticed a group of slim young men jogging on the sand. One of them said hopefully, "Just think, one day we'll be able to run at the beach." The other one laughed out loud and said, "Just think, one day we'll be able to take our shirts off at the beach!"

Spit take

It's no secret that laughter is often touted as "the best medicine." But where does laughter rank when it comes to healing our minds?

If you have ever laughed so hard that you almost peed yourself, chuckled until your cheeks hurt, or even had a case of the uncontrollable church giggles, you might not be surprised to learn that laughter is one of God's greatest gifts when it comes to mental health. That's because you have already experienced the rewarding sensation and sentiment that follows an episode of side-splitting laughter.

Laughter releases endorphins that relieve pain and create an overall sense of well-being. Laughter lowers blood pressure, reduces worry and stress, and boosts the immune system. Laughter is also a powerful weapon against anger and resentment and can usually diffuse a tense or uncomfortable situation.

With all these benefits and no adverse side effects, unless of course Sister Mary Immaculata (who we cleverly nicknamed Sister Mary I'llsmackulota) catches you with the church giggles, you might agree that if you could bottle it and sell it, you'd have a profitable product to pitch on *Shark Tank*.

But here's the giggle: it's free and it is everywhere!

Luckily for our contestants, the laughs are not only gratis and plentiful but par for the course when a group of adults come together on national television to share some of the most intimate details of their lives. They use the absurdity of their situation to laugh continuously and work through some of their most difficult trials.

That's right... hilarity can be found in some of life's most arduous circumstances, because humor is a matter of perspective. When you can look at a situation, especially your own, and find comedy in your predicaments, you are more equipped to face those situations head-on. You'll stop trying to camouflage and conceal them. In fact, when you can see a portion of your life as "funny," you are more likely to share it. And as we already know, sharing an experience of life allows both parties to acquire knowledge, grow, and change for the better.

Doubled over with laughter

Scott and Jordan were teammates and roommates, and although they couldn't have been more different, their love of laughing drew them together, and they were soon inseparable. While on the show, the contestants became addicted to a high-intensity cardio workout known as spinning. It offered them a challenging workout, a way to bond, and a great deal of laughs! The guys decided that in order to look and feel more like professional cyclists, they would need to dress the part, so they placed an order for some brand new spinning garb that soon arrived at the ranch. They were so excited about their package that they bolted upstairs to try on their form-fitting cycle gear. Scott and Jordan got laughing so hard when they saw each other that they decided to share the chuckle with the others. So into the kitchen they pranced in unitards that looked like *Build-A-Bear* had filled the order. The other contestants were falling off their chairs at the sight of two relatively large, grown men stuffed into red and black Lycra tubes that were stretched far beyond their capacity, like trying to fit ten pounds of potatoes into a five-pound sack. We all appreciated and benefited from the shared laugh and were glad they had not kept it to themselves. The image lives rent-free in my head and still generates a giggle whenever I see a spin bike.

Our contestants aren't privy to something unique or unattainable by the general public; they just quickly realize that laughter is essential to navigate and conquer the mental and physical challenges that lie ahead. So surround yourself with people who make you laugh, and if you happen to be the class clown, share that gift with others—their mental health may hinge on it.

> *A cheerful heart is good medicine, but a broken spirit saps a person's strength.*
> —*Proverbs 17:22 (NLT)*

WEIGHING IN

At a young age, I realized how important and contagious laughter was. I've seen a lot of rough things in my life, but one thing that's kept me upbeat and positive despite hardship is laughing and helping others do the same. For me, laughter was a way to see the good instead of focusing on the difficult. Find a way to see what you have gained, not just what you have lost, and you too can not only see the humor in life but also find joy!

Billy Connolly once said, *"Before you judge a man, walk a mile in his shoes. After that who cares?... He's a mile away and you've got his shoes!"*

—Jordan Alicandro, *Former Biggest Loser contestant, Season 16: Glory Days*

Episode 10:
UTILIZE POSITIVE SELF-TALK

Remember as a kid when you would show everyone the things you could do? A somersault, jumping in the pool, or running really, really fast. "Watch this" is every kid's mantra. You wanted everyone to see that you could do it, even if it was just an attempt with no actual results. Why did we do that? Perhaps it was because the world hadn't gotten into our heads and convinced us otherwise. Up until that point, we were proud of anything and everything we attempted, whether we were going to succeed or fail. And we wanted everyone to see that we were something special.

Hang on every word

While working on the show, I found The Canyon Challenge to be one of the most nerve-wracking events ever attempted. In this challenge, the contestants were fitted in full-body harnesses and then hung one hundred feet in the air on a wire that crossed a six-hundred-foot ravine. Their job was to, hand over hand, pull themselves from one side of the canyon to the other while their legs dangled over the massive gorge. As the blue team made their way across the canyon, I noticed that Damien, the only man on the team, was speaking words of encouragement to each of his terrified female teammates as they struggled to pull their body weight over the pass.

Up first was Gina, a former cheerleader from Texas, who was sweeter than stolen honey and, at this moment, as nervous as a fly in a glue pot. As she scrambled to make her way along the treacherous wire, Damien led the cheer with a bevy of heartfelt supportive words to embolden and keep her from giving up. Although a former NFL lineman, perfectly capable of having his booming voice reverberate throughout the valley, Damien simply leaned in and gently reminded her to "Be aggressive, B-E aggressive!" In addition, he assured her: "You got this, baby girl." "You're stronger than you know." "You can do anything." "You're gonna make your kids so proud." And "you got more guts than you can hang on a fence" in an attempt to make her feel at home.

Next in line to make the pass was Lori, a three-time Olympic gold medal softball pitcher. But there was nothing soft about her game. She was one of the most fearless competitors I had ever met. When she hit the wire, Damien's demeanor and volume quickly changed to match his teammate's need to outplay, outwork, and outlast her competition. Now he was barking his messages of motivation: "You are the strongest woman here." "You are fearless." "Don't you dare give up on yourself." And a few "put your ass in gear!" just for good measure.

Damien knew exactly what each of those ladies needed to hear in order to make it across that ravine.

Wouldn't it be nice if we knew how to talk to ourselves? If we knew how to encourage and celebrate and love ourselves? The world has a way of taking that ability from us. If you hear "you can't do that" enough, you'll start to believe it. In fact, you will start telling yourself that very thing.

We need to change the way we are talking to ourselves because words, especially the ones we tell ourselves, hold incredible power. But positive self-talk doesn't always come easy, mostly because we have been living in the lies that others have dumped on us over and over again throughout our lives: You're not good enough, you aren't worth it, you won't win. These lies make us feel unworthy and unlovable and make it very difficult to believe that we are capable of greatness.

Damien's ability to speak the very words of encouragement that each of his teammates needed in that moment might be because he has seven children and is likely very practiced in knowing what each child needs to hear when they have an obstacle to overcome. You know who else knows how to speak words of love and affirmation to each of His children? I'll give you a second here...

The next time you hear a voice in your head telling you, you can't, you're weak, you're unworthy, or any other nonsense, do yourself a favor and stop listening! Instead, direct your attention to what God is saying because He is the one who made you and therefore teaches you to say, "I praise you because I am fearfully and wonderfully made; Your works are wonderful, I know that full well." (Psalm 139:14, NIV)

Put in a good word

My daughter works for a party princess company here in SoCal. Various storybook royalty are hired to be special guests at birthday parties and other celebrations. While at the party, the princess will sing, dance, tell stories, and oversee her court's royal twirls and waves, but what makes this party company unique is that all of the princesses guide their young attendees through a series of affirmations. They teach them to recite: "I am loved. I am confident. I am strong. I am brave. I am chosen by God to do something amazing in this world." Imagine if that is how we spoke to ourselves every day. Oh, the things we could accomplish! Now get this, each of those statements is a truth about you. Yes, you! Even if you don't feel they are one hundred percent verifiable at this moment. Creating a mantra and reminding yourself of these truths is a great way to start believing them. So you can crash a few princess parties to see the benefits of life-affirming words or simply write your personal attestations and post them on your bathroom mirror to read daily. You can record yourself speaking words of truth and set them as your alarm, enlist them as your screensaver, sing them loud and proud in your car, or even announce them in a royal proclamation. Whatever you decide, start using words to remind yourself what God already knows: You were chosen to do something amazing in this world.

Words are alive, and when we speak them into the universe, they have power. The power to hurt but also the power to heal. Remember in the beginning, everything that God created He first spoke.

*"And God said, "Let there be light"; and there was light.
And God saw that the light was good;" —Genesis 1:3-4*

Everything that He created is good, and each is preceded by words that are good. If we focus on His words, trust them, and ultimately believe them, then we can tumble and dive, win the race, cross any ravine, and be proud of our accomplishments. "Because it is only when we have the faith of a child that we will then have the strength of a man."[xvi]

Hey, God, watch this!

WEIGHING IN

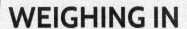

Trust me, from someone who's weighed 322 pounds and has lost over 160 pounds and kept it off, changing your negative self-talk into positive self-talk takes time.

It's a habit we have to unlearn. Learning it didn't happen overnight and neither will unlearning it. To me, positive self-talk is like a muscle. Just like in fitness, you have to constantly flex that muscle in order to REALLY see it come through, especially in the beginning stages. The more you work it, the less you have to "flex." One day, that muscle will be so big and prominent, you won't need to flex... it's just there.

The definition of insanity is doing the same thing over and over and expecting a different result, right? So why not change the narrative. Turn your internal dialogue to FM (For Me) stations vs. AM (Against Me) stations. Any time you talk to yourself poorly, write it down. Ask why do I talk to myself that way, and how is this serving me?

The more you work it, the easier it becomes.

—**Erica Lugo,** *Trainer on The Biggest Loser 2020 and founder and owner of EricaFitLove*

Episode 11:
NEVER STOP LEARNING

An intelligent mind acquires knowledge, and the ear of the wise seeks knowledge.
—*Proverbs 18:15*

Our contestants are no strangers to change. They experience change in some way, shape, or form daily. The most amazing thing about change is that all change offers with it an opportunity to learn. When you continue to nourish your mind with information and the development of new skills, you will inevitably boost your level of self-efficacy, or simply your belief in your own abilities to rise to challenges and successfully complete tasks.

I have seen firsthand how cultivating self-efficacy directly affects outcomes when contestants are faced with challenges, giving them the confidence to succeed. Continued learning allows you to feel more competent, which naturally leads to increased confidence. And when that happens, the possibilities are boundless.

One afternoon, as Scott and I sat together for lunch, he encouraged me to try, as he often did, one of his culinary creations. Today's special was a tuna fish and blueberry sandwich. We called it a tuna-fruity! It was there I realized that Scott was becoming increasingly and somewhat overconfident in his newly acquired cooking skills. But, unlike the sandwich, that wasn't necessarily a bad thing. In fact, a great deal of Scott's weight-loss journey was about rebuilding his confidence through the lessons he was learning. And he soon found that these life-changing lessons could offer others support and guidance on their voyage of healing as well.

Working knowledge

Following his retirement from the NFL, Scott had often entertained the idea of working as a sports commentator, but due to a limited belief in his ability, he had narrowed his own vision. His time on the ranch gave him a clearer understanding of what actually brought him joy and taught him to chase his dreams. So following his disappointing elimination from the show, he enrolled himself in broadcasting school and learned how to fulfill what he had always envisioned. He found purpose and power behind his experiences and his new script on life. When he was bold enough to combine his life lessons with humor, hope, encouragement, and, of course, sports, he found a platform that allowed him to reach others in ways that limiting himself would have never permitted.

It is by living and learning, healing and sharing that we can serve others by offering them the space and resources to heal as well. And that's exactly what he set out to do. Today Scott hosts a sports talk radio show called *Unrivaled*, where he takes an entertaining and insightful look at sports. Through his show, he continues to inspire, encourage, and motivate his listeners. The learning process opened his eyes to what brought him pain and what brought him joy. And once he knew the difference, his choices in life became easy.

There is endless happiness and healing in continued learning because that is how we discover all we are capable of and how God will use our knowledge, our skill, talent, and life stories to serve Him best.

WEIGHING IN

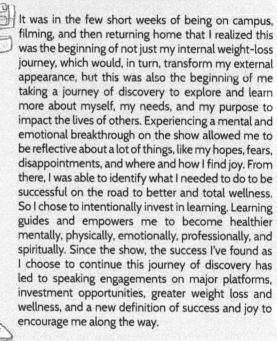

It was in the few short weeks of being on campus, filming, and then returning home that I realized this was the beginning of not just my internal weight-loss journey, which would, in turn, transform my external appearance, but this was also the beginning of me taking a journey of discovery to explore and learn more about myself, my needs, and my purpose to impact the lives of others. Experiencing a mental and emotional breakthrough on the show allowed me to be reflective about a lot of things, like my hopes, fears, disappointments, and where and how I find joy. From there, I was able to identify what I needed to do to be successful on the road to better and total wellness. So I chose to intentionally invest in learning. Learning guides and empowers me to become healthier mentally, physically, emotionally, professionally, and spiritually. Since the show, the success I've found as I choose to continue this journey of discovery has led to speaking engagements on major platforms, investment opportunities, greater weight loss and wellness, and a new definition of success and joy to encourage me along the way.

"No matter where you are in life, celebrate it. It's either the product of your growth or the place that will help you grow."

—**Ms. PhiXavier Holmes,** *former contestant, The Biggest Loser 2020*

SEASON FINALE:
MIND

We have just discussed seven keys to unlocking, healing, and promoting the health of our minds:

- being intentional when we set out to attain a goal
- forming a network of peers who are working toward the same objective
- allowing the movement of our body to fuel our mind
- being more conscious of ourselves and the world around us
- engaging in more laughter
- speaking words of kindness and affirmation
- engaging in lifelong learning

Touchdown!

Scott discovered that his mind needed healing before his physical self was willing to cooperate. And when his mind found a path to being well, his body followed suit and his true self emerged and prevailed. His pilgrimage was marred with affliction, but from his days of playing football, Scott recognized this truth:

> "We rejoice in our sufferings, knowing that suffering produces endurance, and endurance produces character, and character produces hope, and hope does not disappoint us"
> —Romans 5:3–5.

Which of the seven strategies can you implement today to help heal your mind and bring you one step closer to wellness and living your very best life?

Season 4

SOUL

Sonya's Story

The body apart from the spirit is dead
—James 2:26

In one of my earliest days working on *The Biggest Loser*, we were in the gym filming what is referred to as the "first chance" workout. Not only was it the initial workout of the season, but it was also my first experience with the contestants. Now if you can, imagine a group of gravely overweight participants, most with serious health issues, some who had never set foot in a gym, and still others who completely lacked the physical and mental ability to make it through the next hour. In this workout, they would abruptly be pushed to and beyond their physical and mental limits, with cameras literally in their faces. It is entirely possible that I was just as, if not more so, terrified than the contestants.

So there I was with a blood pressure cuff in one hand and a puke bucket in the other. (Working on TV is incredibly glamorous!) I was standing just off-camera when I noticed one of the contestants in a remote corner of the gym, all by herself, pushing through a series of step-ups onto a box that seemed to rival her in height. I noticed that with every step she took, she recited a short phrase that seemed to be propelling her legs up and onto the box.

My curiosity got the best of me, so I moved in closer to get a better sense of what was transpiring in that corner and, of course, to make sure that her blood pressure hadn't spiked, causing her to be loopy. But as I approached and landed within earshot, my brain began to process what she was saying, and instantly my heart burst wide open, my eyes welled, and tears spilled over the rims onto my cheeks. This five-foot-four-inch 283-pound woman was reaffirming with every breath she took "With Him, all things are possible!"

And it was precisely in that moment that I realized, without Him, what we were attempting to do here was completely impossible!

Just to be clear, when I say Him, I am, of course, referring to God, not any of our handsome trainers. Although on the set, those two tend to get a bit confused!

The soul is the aspect of ourselves that can carry us through anything. When our legs fail and our mind quits, it is our soul that carries us from one side to the other, as was evidenced by my dear friend Sonya from season 16. Her mantra in the gym that day enabled me to see that God needed to be a central part of this considerable life-changing journey, or the participants would never fully heal and would continue struggling to attain wellness.

The human soul is God within us. However, the human soul is often the most neglected part of ourselves because we fail to realize our souls need attention in order to foster healing and attain wellness. Just as we fuel our bodies and exercise our minds, we, too, need to nurture our souls through purposeful practices, prayer, and passion.

> *Bless the Lord, O my soul; and all that is within me, bless his holy name.*
> *—Psalm 103:1*

This section of the book will remind you of, and in some cases introduce you to, seven practices that will make your soul a priority and keep it in shape so you can continue working toward wellness and experience all that it has to offer.

Episode 12:

HUMILITY

We learn humility through accepting humiliations cheerfully.
—Mother Teresa

Sonya was getting packed for her journey to The Biggest Loser ranch when she decided that she would probably need a bathing suit. After all, she was headed to sunny Southern California. So she rifled through her drawers and located a swimsuit that hadn't seen the light of day in years. Just to make sure it still fit and would be acceptable on national television, she tried it on in the privacy of her bedroom. "Not too shabby," she thought, until she noticed that her cat, who had been watching the fashion show, vomited and walked out of the room. This painfully humbling experience provided a huge benefit on her journey because humility is the first step in healing your soul.

The tranquility of humility

Being humble allows you to see your intrinsic worth, not what the world would suggest makes you worthy. Just as importantly, humility reminds you that there is a power greater than yourself, and it's this gentle reminder that allows you to relinquish control to that higher power.

God is in control. Remember, He is the one who made us—perfectly and wonderfully. Yet, even though we are perfectly made, do we abuse our physical and mental selves and then not like what we see? Does our reflection feel less than perfect? Yes, of course... that happens to all of us. But humility takes us out of our own pity party and self-judgement and reminds us that God doesn't see us the same way the world sees us or the way that we often see ourselves. He sees us as His magnificent child. He accepts us as we truly are—perfect. When we are humble enough to accept ourselves as we truly are, we shed all of the expectations that society puts on us. God loves us simply because we are His. By accepting who we are and abdicating ultimate authority to God, we will begin to heal our souls.

My husband has been an AA sponsor for years after his own personal battle with alcohol. (But that is a whole separate book.) To help his new sponsees, he often brings them to our alluring surf and asks them if they believe there is a higher power to which they can surrender. Inevitably, one of them will say no because addicts, more often than not, feel the need to be in control. That's when my husband encourages them to step into the turbulent Pacific to see how long it takes before a massive wave knocks them down. Whether you want to believe it or not, there is something more powerful in this world than you. Humility is recognizing that you cannot take on the world alone; you need God's help and to remember that God's way is better than the world's way.

> *The world tells us to seek success, power and money;*
> *God tells us to seek humility, service and love.*
> —*Pope Francis*

Recipe for great-tasting humble pie

We live in a relatively self-centered society, so humility doesn't come naturally for most of us. The good news is that humility, just like any other practice, can be nurtured and developed with a few simple strategies. Implement these eight challenges today and every day to experience and benefit from the gift of humility.

Got help?

By auditioning for the show, our contestants are acknowledging "my way is no longer working." They are asking for help. It takes a brave person to admit they can't do something on their own and that their way isn't necessarily the right way. The words "I need help" don't usually come easy, but they always come with a huge reward, especially in the humility department.

Cruise control

Accepting help is a huge step towards humility, unless you continue dictating the terms of the assistance. Allowing others to bail you out or give a hand up without your self-imposed restriction is a leap of faith that fosters humility.

Share your inner DIIP

Share your deficiencies, imperfections, insecurities, and problems with compassionate ears. Support groups are an easy way to practice transparency and continue to grow in humility.

I beg your pardon

Failure is inevitable because we are human and, therefore, fallible. When we seek forgiveness, we are revealing that we have failed, but it's in that disclosure that we encounter humility. "I'm sorry" are the two most humbling and healing words in history. Use them abundantly!

At your service

Every time we put others' needs before our own, we are becoming increasingly humble. Rick Warren says that "humility is not thinking less of yourself, it's thinking of yourself less."

STAN-down

We all know the person that can't help but "one up" everyone else. We call that person STAN (Sh*t! That Ain't Nothin'). Humility comes when you are willing to concede and take a backseat instead of trying to outdo someone else's story.

Ears open, mouth shut, hand up

Social media platforms have convinced us that everything we have to say is of the utmost importance, but they are wrong. Very little of what we say has value because, honestly, no one is paying attention. We are all too busy talking and trying to be heard. Taking a step back and listening to those around us and asking questions to better understand another's point of view will quickly win us favor and help us practice humility. Talk and post less, listen more!

What's your shoe size?

It's one thing to be sympathetic, to feel sorry for someone, but quite another to be empathetic. Empathy is the ability to understand and share the feeling of another human being. Placing yourself in another person's shoes is a surefire way to gain a better appreciation of what they're going through. When you understand and truly feel another person's pain, you will easily be humbled.

Understanding and practicing humility gives you the ability to accept yourself as you truly are—the good, the bad, the beautiful, the ugly, the success, and the failure... all of it. Accept that this is you and that you are made in the image and likeness of God Almighty. And if you don't like the person looking back at you in the mirror, relinquish that to God because He is more powerful than you, and it is by loving Him first that we can begin to love ourselves. Humbling yourself to Him is the first step in healing your soul. Like Mother Teresa reminds us, "If you are really humble, if you realize how small you are and how much you need God, then you cannot fail."

Humble yourselves before the Lord, and he will exalt you.
—James 4:10

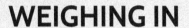

WEIGHING IN

When we start our days as St. Augustine did, "praying as though everything depends on God and working as though everything depends on us," we are living humbly in the presence of Christ.

That doesn't mean that our days won't be filled with challenges and, sometimes, even hardships. For those moments, I offer you a simple prayer that will embolden and fortify you to abide in His company so that you are capable of living fully and freely every moment of every day.

"God grant me the serenity to accept the things I cannot change, courage to change the things I can, and wisdom to know the difference."

—**Matthew Tennison**, *MD CAQSM FACEP, Department of Emergency Medicine, UNM School of Medicine associate professor, assistant sports medicine fellowship director, assistant team physician at UNM Lobos, physician on The Biggest Loser 2020*

Episode 13:
PRAYER, SILENCE, AND SAINTS

Are any of you suffering hardships? You should pray.
—James 5:13 (NLT)

"Now I lay me down to sleep, a bag of peanuts at my feet. If I die before I wake, give them to my Uncle Jake."

That was my favorite prayer when I was a kid, not because it had any redemptive value or because I was excited about the windfall Uncle Jake would receive should I croak in the night. It was my favorite prayer because my Grandpa Knopp taught it to me and would recite it at the foot of my bed.

Pray tell

Prayer has the power to mend broken souls. My grandpa carried around the weight of a broken soul for most of his life, but in those brief moments of prayer at the foot of my bed, he was standing with God.

Prayer heals not because of the flowery, poetic words we string together to impress God as they effortlessly roll off our tongue. Prayer heals our souls because through prayer, we abandon ourselves, the noise, and the distractions of the world to become one with Him. We stand at the foot of the bed in the presence of God Almighty.

The earnest prayer of a righteous person has great power
and produces wonderful results.
—James 5:16 (NLT)

Amen to that

As a lifelong Catholic, I recognize that, just like people, prayer comes in all shapes and sizes, but all effective prayer has one thing in common: it can change hearts and heal souls. My prayer life has developed over the years, and I have found various prayer practices that support and mature my relationship with God. For one, I am a huge advocate of praying the rosary. I actually fell in love with the rosary driving back and forth through the treacherous Los Angeles traffic, praying for the stunt performers that I work with in various live shows at Universal Studios Hollywood. This practice alone has brought me incredible peace and purpose as I reflect on the decades, revealing important events in the life, death, and resurrection of Christ through the eyes of His beloved Mother. You can pray the rosary in so many ways, and it never gets boring. I can't think of a better way to spend twenty minutes a day with God. If it has been years since you have picked up your rosary, I highly suggest you give it a whirl; you will be amazed at the promises it holds.

Though formal prayer is great, not all prayers have to be formal. The nuns used to tell us that singing to God counts as praying twice, and not wanting to miss out on a bargain, I have taken that counsel to heart. I love worship music and use it often to let God know just how much I love Him (although with my lack of pitch, tone, and rhythm, He might not see it that way). One of my favorite memories from season 16 was sneaking Sonya off the ranch and into downtown Los Angeles on her fortieth birthday. That day she fulfilled a lifelong dream of attending Hillsong Church and being surrounded in the glory of God through their dynamic live worship music. It was glorious and liberating to raise our hands and voices in praise of His beautiful name, and one look at the pure joy pouring out of Sonya that day told you unequivocally that worship music is a powerful form of prayer.

Like most of us, if your phone is preventing you from folding your hands in prayer, might I suggest a way to make your new appendage a part of your worship team? You have so many great resources for daily prayer available right at your fingertips. It's like carrying around a little church in your hand.

⊕ The "Pray As You Go" app—offers ten–twelve-minute prayer sessions based on the daily readings, with insightful questions to help you start conversations with God. Plus, each of their readers has a soothing accent or a lilting brogue, always a bonus in my book! This app is free of charge.

⊕ "Hallow"—offers a wealth of guided meditations, prayer challenges, and fosters praying in our fast-paced world. Prayer sessions can be tailored to your time constraints, making any time the right time to spend with God. This app requires a monthly or annual fee, but they offer a free trial.

⊕ "Formed"—you can watch, read, and listen to engaging Catholic content on demand. There is a small fee, but some parishes gift the access code to their parishioners. Check if your church is one of them.

⊕ The "Laudate" app—the #1 Catholic app is jam-packed with great Catholic resources. My favorites include the interactive rosary and the examination of conscience to refer to while in the confessional. The app is free and available on the Apple App Store and Google Play.

⊕ The "Reimagining The Examen" app—a wonderful tool that guides you in reviewing, repenting, and resolving the events of the day. This app is also free.

⊕ Rosary podcasts are plentiful and offer numerous choices to lead you in prayer and reflection. However, if you are more of a visual person, you can find several rosary series on YouTube that showcase awe-inspiring works of art depicting the various scenes in the life of Christ. My favorite series is offered by Kate and Mike Catholic Crusade.

Gone are the days of reciting only the handful of devotions we learned in school; there is something for everyone when it comes to deepening our relationship with God. But remember, talking to God is only half of it.

Shhh!

The other half is listening to what He has to say to you. But in this world of constant noise, it is almost impossible to hear the voice of God. That is why the second part of prayer is finding silence. For it is in that silence that you will hear His voice. As Keating tells us, "Silence is God's first language; everything else is just a poor translation."

One of the greatest honors of my life was having the privilege to speak about the impact that The Mass Journal has had on our family in a Dynamic Catholic promotional video. In the video, we present the idea that we so often teach our kids to listen to their coaches, teachers, priests, and other adults, but we have simply forgotten to teach them to listen to the voice of God. The voice that will lead them, guide them, and heal them—because it is in His whispers that we will hear blessings and receive grace.

The importance of silence cannot be overstated. And one of the hidden bonuses that our contestants receive on their weight-loss journey is the gift of silence. There are no phones, computers, TVs, radios, mail, or newspapers on our campus. Now, granted, this doesn't scream sign me up, but it is something that our contestants tell us they actually miss when they go back home. I know that for a good deal of them, it is in that silence that they were encouraged, directed, and strengthened by the words of God.

Prayer and silence are instrumental in healing the soul. A routine of daily prayer and moments of silence are just what the soul doctor ordered.

Dear St. Anthony, come around...

Over the years, I have found enormous strength and encouragement in my prayer life by leaning into the saints and the lessons they offer in developing a prayerful relationship with God. The saints are our friends in heaven, and just as we would ask our friends here on Earth to pray with and for us, we petition the saints to do the same. They are exemplary Christians that reside in heaven with the Lord Almighty and, through their extraordinary lives, show us how we can be changed for the better when we turn to God in prayer, and how the healing of our souls comes from giving ourselves over to Him completely. So when I go to work to physically heal a body, I bring the saints along to guide me in healing the soul.

Many of the stuntmen and women that I work with carry St. Genesius medals that I have administered to them in times of need. He is the patron of performers, actors, and comedians, so I naturally assigned my stunt performers to him as well. It was through a very public act of prayer that St. Genesius's soul was cleansed, and he felt, for the first time, the presence of God.

The dancers that I work with often receive St. Vitus medals, and the athletes, St. Sebastian. And, of course, St. Anthony is called upon whenever losing is a problem, including losing ball games.

St. Charles Borromeo, the patron saint of the overweight and dieters, is the saint that comes with me on set. Because of his tenacity and persistence against the enemies of the church, St. Charles Borromeo was instrumental in the reform of the Catholic Church. He reminds us to turn to God for the strength needed to fight our battles, especially when our battles are self-inflicted. God used him to show us that change for the better is possible, even against immeasurable odds. His medallions can often be found by our contestants' bedsides or in their pockets during a workout.

The saints have guided me in conversation with God throughout my life. Their intercessions have supplied me with strength and courage and emboldened me to be with Christ in all that I do daily. I once heard these words by a very wise man, and I try to live by them myself: "The key to a life of prayer is to place your shoes far under your bed every night. That way you are forced to your knees every morning before you attempt the day." I believe this man and my Grandpa Knopp would have been fast friends.

A soul arms itself by prayer for all kinds of combat. In whatever state the soul may be, it ought to pray. A soul

which is pure and beautiful must pray, or else it will
lose its beauty; a soul which is striving after this purity
must pray, or else it will never attain it; a soul which is
newly converted must pray, or else it will fall again; a
sinful soul, plunged in sins, must pray so that it might rise
again. There is no soul which is not bound to pray, for
every single grace comes to the soul through prayer.
—St. Faustina

WEIGHING IN

As I mentioned above, The Mass Journal is a great way
to record what God is saying to us in the Mass, through
prayer and in silence. Throughout the process of
writing this book, I flipped back through the pages of
my old Mass Journals (a tip recommended by Matthew
Kelly) looking for inspiration when I was lacking it and
encouragement when I was ready to give up. There in
my little handwritten books, I found a treasure trove of
lessons, advice, and insight, all from the mouth of God! I
heard God speaking them into my heart, so I jotted them
down, but at the time, I didn't realize that I would need so
many of those words to move forward with this project. I
remembered that God isn't late or early. God is always on
time, as are the words and gifts He shares with us. Mass
journals are a great way to hold onto all the wisdom He
sends our way for the time we need it most. You can grab
any little notepad to use as a mass journal, or you can
order The Mass Journal at DynamicCatholic.com. They
are free; you simply pay for shipping! They have become
a spiritual practice for our family, and I hope they will
become a part of your prayer and silence as well.

—Kelly

Episode 14:
LET GO

In season 16's episode "The End Zone" and season 17's episode "The Final Cut," the remaining contestants were fitted with multiple sandbags equaling the amount of weight they had lost throughout the season. The objective for each challenge was to navigate the course (e.g., around a stadium or up a steep climb) while shedding the weighted bags at each of the drop zones. The ultimate goal of the challenge was to come across the finish line free from the burdens that were holding them back at the beginning of the race.

It's not too far of a leap to see the hidden message in this type of a challenge. In order to successfully move forward, you have to let go of the things that are weighing you down.

Take it or leave it

Luis and his twin brother, Roberto, were a force to be reckoned with on *The Biggest Loser: Temptation Nation*. Roberto was one of the top three competitors for the $250,000 grand prize, and Luis was the front-runner for the at-home prize of $100,000. So finale week for the Hernandez family was not only incredibly exciting but also exceptionally stressful.

A few days before the finale, I found Luis in his hotel room reeling with anxiety and fear. He was physically and mentally exhausted, and the stress of winning at all costs was taking a huge toll on his soul. He was not behaving like the same sweet man I had grown so fond of on the ranch. I tried for hours to talk him down and ease his unrest but wasn't making any progress... until I remembered that healing is found when you hand over your pain, your fears, your disappointments, and your anger to Christ. So I pulled him out of his room (much easier to do after having lost 134 pounds) and marched him across the street to a little church I had seen when I parked that morning. There I told him he needed to shed it all at the foot of the cross and we were not leaving this little church until it was securely in Christ's hands. That way he could successfully move forward whether he was about to win or lose. In one of the more beautiful moments I had the privilege to share with a contestant, I watched this man who seemed so heavy-hearted reluctantly pull himself to the altar and leave behind the burdens that were weighing him down. When he turned around to leave the church, it was evident that God was there with His arms open wide, eager to bear the weight of Luis's sandbags.

The burdens we carry are many, but Christ has given us the greatest gift possible: the ability to leave our sins, our brokenness, our pain, our pride, our fears, our failures... all of it, with Him. It is He who takes that from us so we can continue to move forward, allowing our battered and broken souls to heal and open our lives to joy.

Don't hold on to anything. There is nothing you are holding on to that is safer in your hands than in God's.
—Dr. Greg Bottaro, *The Mindful Catholic*

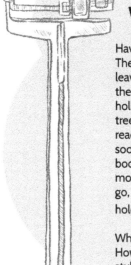

WEIGHING IN

Have you ever heard how a hunter catches a monkey? The hunter will take a coconut and hollow out the inside, leaving a hole just big enough for a monkey's hand. Then the hunter will place a piece of sweet fruit inside the hollowed-out coconut. He then ties the coconut to a tree. The monkey, upon smelling the tropical treat, will reach inside the coconut and grab hold of his jackpot, but soon realizes that he cannot fit both his hand and the booty back through the tiny hole. Luckily for the hunter, monkeys are incredibly stubborn, and instead of letting go, withdrawing his hand, and moving on, the monkey holds tight and becomes easy prey for the hunter. [xvii]

When we refuse to let go, we become easy prey. However, when we release the things that we are stubbornly holding on to, we will always be rewarded with the real prize: freedom.

—Kelly

Episode 15:
SACRED MOMENTS

As a woman in her fifties who has asked her fair share of questions, I have come to fully agree with one of history's most compelling characters, Don Juan, who, in the 1994 film entitled Don Juan DeMarco, reminds us, "There are only four questions of value in life... What is sacred? Of what is the spirit made? What is worth living for, and what is worth dying for? The answer to each is the same."

Just like in algebra, if we simply figure out the answer to the first question, we are then capable of identifying the others and have then discovered the answer to life's most paramount questions. So what is sacred? Well here's the kicker: for each of us, the answer will be completely different.

Divine intervention

Let me share with you how I came to figure out "what is sacred" for myself. Years ago, I was sitting at the computer for what seemed like hours, trying to find the perfect definition of the word sacred for a presentation I was tasked with at work, when my then-seven-year-old son innocently approached and asked what I was doing.

"I'm Googling." (If we are going to be honest, by this point, I was on Gizoogle, so I could see what sacred meant to... well... Snoop Dog?) Then my sweet Danny offered that he knew what it meant. And as any loving mother would, I said, "Oh for goodness' sake, humor me." And this child, without hesitation, said, "Sacred is when something touches you so deeply inside that you can never describe it with words, and sometimes it even makes you better." True story!

As I sat there in shock and amazement, I thought, Isn't he the same kid who just cut holes in his brand new jeans for ventilation? Yet he so eloquently, and from his heart, expressed what I had been trying to define and label for hours. Instead of defining sacred with words, it needs to be experienced in the moments of our life.

As you can imagine, we have lots of sacred moments on *The Biggest Loser*. Throughout my time on the show, I have had hundreds of interactions that I would certainly consider sacred, but none touched my soul as much as this one moment.

Prior to the final casting cuts, we were administering a swim test for each of the potential contestants, just to make sure that they were capable of participating in any water-related events if they were to be cast on the show. We didn't know the potential contestants at this point, as this was our first real interaction with the group. One at a time, the participants entered the pool area, jumped in, swam the length of the pool, trod water, and then climbed out. The next participant up was a young man, so as he strode across the deck, I asked him to remove his shirt and stand at the edge of the pool. He reluctantly pulled off his shirt and headed to the deep end. When he didn't jump in right away, I asked if he could swim. He said yes, but he was visibly shaken. So I asked what had him so distraught. As he choked back tears, he divuldged, "I had a sex change operation nine years ago, and since then, I have not taken my shirt off in public. Besides my wife, you are the only person who has ever seen my scars." Honestly, his self-consciousness was unwarranted, as I hadn't noticed his scars. But what I did notice was an overwhelming sense of connection that drew me to comfort him.

There we were, a fifty-year-old woman and a 400-pound transgender man, complete strangers, standing embraced at the edge of the pool with tears running down both of our cheeks. His pain was palpable, and I was desperate to somehow alleviate it, but all I knew how to do was to hold him. That moment was sacred. It touched me so deeply that I will never be able to describe it with words, and it truly made me better than I was moments before. In that embrace, I knew that God was healing both of our souls because it is when we care for

98

each other as God cares for us that we get to truly experience what is sacred. And when you are aware of the sacred moments in your life, you will feel the presence of Christ. He will be right there healing your soul.

> *We are always in the presence of God. There is never a non-sacred moment! His presence never diminishes. Our awareness of His presence may falter, but the reality of His presence never changes.*
> —Max Lucado

When we are vulnerable enough to reveal ourselves to God, any moment can become a sacred moment. It's our job to recognize that they are sacred and to live in them, even if it is just for that moment. And I can promise you this: You are never the same person following a sacred moment that you were before. They will always change you for the better.

WEIGHING IN

In the first episode of the season, we were tasked with running a one-mile course in which, much to my humiliation, I finished at the end of the pack. From there, things only got worse. Each challenge that I lost left me feeling discouraged and defeated, and the thought of failing again became downright daunting. As a former football player and now a coach, I have always been a competitor, so the fact that I kept losing was especially difficult.

But the final challenge of the season changed everything. This time it was a redemption run to see if we had improved on our mile times. After months of caring for my body, preparing my mind, and healing my soul, I am happy to report that I shaved eight minutes off my mile and won the challenge! When I crossed the finish line, for the first time in a long time, I knew that I could hold my head high and that my wife and sons would be especially proud of me. That moment was truly a sacred moment. Not because I had won but because I had improved and, through those improvements, had made my loved ones proud. Being an example for my family is what I hold most sacred. And that is my "why" every day to staying healthy.

—Jim Dibattista, winner of *The Biggest Loser* 2020

Episode 16:
GRATITUDE

Gracious words are a honeycomb, sweet to the soul and healing to the bones.
—Proverbs 16:24 (NIV)

Teri had every reason to be frustrated, sullen, and angry. She was nearly through the show and had been making great strides toward being one of the season's top competitors. She had already lost thirty-eight pounds, made several advances toward a healthier lifestyle, and rediscovered her true love, swimming. Her time in the pool reminded her that the sport she once loved could provide her body with the exercise it needed to heal her mind, restoring the peace and quiet it had been searching for. In addition, Teri says that the smell of a pool has the power to take you back to your childhood. I agree, and often, we find healing in that alone.

Then it happened: during one of the weekly challenges, Teri jumped feet first into a shallow mud pit and fractured her fibula. With a walking boot and instructions to not bear weight for the next eight weeks, it seemed like Teri was definitely out of the running and would be heading home soon. But much to our surprise, Teri did not give up so easily. I have been working in sports medicine for over twenty-five years, and she was by far the greatest comeback story I have ever witnessed. It was all because of her commitment to an attitude of gratitude.

There wasn't a moment that Teri didn't express gratitude for the things that she was capable of doing and for the people who were working to accommodate her new disability. She never complained about what she couldn't do, but instead showed gratitude in the gym for the activities that she could participate in and sometimes for the ones she couldn't. In fact, she was incredibly grateful that burpees are contraindicated for fibular fractures! Teri could have gone head-to-head with any of the other contestants in non-weight bearing exercises, and honestly, I would have put my money on her every time.

Instead of being frustrated about her injury and subsequent restrictions, she expressed appreciation to the medical staff for having her best interests in mind, even when the decisions we made were not what she wanted to hear and kept her from fully participating. Without grousing or grumbling, she relied on her new friends to make her meals and wait on her when she was not capable of doing things for herself. Instead of being bitter or letting her ego get in the way, she just showered them with gratitude.

In addition, she was eternally grateful for her ability to swim and her innate love of the water because she knew that it was in the water that her body and her mind could heal and become stronger for the journey ahead. Little did she know that her soul was experiencing that same healing through her constant gratitude.

Goodness gracious!

Gratitude changes everything! A gracious heart affects every aspect of life and directly impacts happiness and mental health.

Gracious people tend to be more optimistic, less self-centered, have increased self-esteem, and strongly believe they can accomplish their goals.

Gratitude affects our mind and our mental state. People who are gracious are less stressed and anxious, more resilient and relaxed, and experience more good feelings and memories.

It has also been found that gratitude leads to better relationships, stronger marriages, and deeper and more fulfilling friendships.

And gratitude even plays a role in our physical health. Those that practice gratitude have stronger immune systems, sleep better, are sick less often, have more energy, and live longer.

And get this: gratitude can also determine your paycheck. People who appreciate the glass being half full have improved networking skills, increased productivity, and improved decision making and management skills, and tend to make more money than people who grumble because the glass is half empty. [xviii]

In fact, Zig Ziglar says that "gratitude is the healthiest of all human emotions." Sound too good to be true? Well, numerous studies have shown that people who keep gratitude journals are overall healthier and happier than those who don't. [xix] Gratitude affects every aspect of life and directly impacts the health of the whole person.

Attitude of gratitude

It seems simple enough, doesn't it? Drop a thank you note, crack a smile, keep a journal. All easy enough to implement into our daily lives, yet gratitude too often gets lost in the busyness of our days and the chaos of our lives. Establishing an attitude of gratitude takes a little bit of effort, but once you get the hang of it, it will make you feel so good you won't want to live without it. To help you make the most of giving and receiving gratitude, follow these tips:

⊕ Write letters or call people from your past and let them know that they have made a difference in your life.

⊕ Be aware of yourself or others complaining and flip the conversation to one with a more positive outcome.

⊕ Surround yourself with the beauty and majesty of nature. It's easy to count your blessings when you are in the middle of them.

⊕ Be in the moment. The past is gone and the future isn't here yet. Gratitude allows you to enjoy the moment you are in.

⊕ Reward effort versus results. Be appreciative of the attempt.

⊕ Set a gratitude timer and find one thing to be grateful for every time the alarm goes off.

⊕ Look at mistakes as opportunities to learn, grow, and be wiser next time.

⊕ Post with a gracious heart. There is too much negativity on social media. Take the opportunity to share gratitude and its many benefits with the world; we all desperately need it.

I once read that "gratitude is God's gift to us." I was certain there had been a misprint. Surely, it was something that we do for Him. But as I watched Teri incorporate gratitude into every part of her day, I realized the truth in that simple statement. Gratitude doesn't change Him; it changes us! Living with a gracious heart and expressing that gratitude through words and actions allows us to live life to the fullest, even in the midst of pain and discomfort.

Teri reminded me that gratitude makes us bulletproof. It is God's armor against the inevitable trials and tribulations in our lives, and yes, it is His healing gift to us.

WEIGHING IN

One of the most harmful addictions, in my opinion, is destination addiction. It's when we say, I'll be happy when I have the perfect job, or the perfect partner, or the perfect body. It is a preoccupation that happiness is somewhere else. When we say, "I'll be happy when..." we are basically telling ourselves that we're not happy right now. Trust me, I spent a lot of my life seeking happiness in external things. Despite success in jobs and good income, I still felt like I was lacking something—no matter what my next "destination" was. It wasn't until I turned inward that I realized happiness is an inside job. It's like looking at a map in a mall and reading the arrow that indicates, "You are here." Well, that's where happiness is. Right here. Any of us can have access to it. The key to unlocking it? Gratitude. Once I started counting my blessings instead of my problems, I realized just how good my life actually is. Once I became thankful for my failures (not just victories), I realized they weren't failures, but rather lessons that made me stronger. The moment I started listening to my inner voice instead of the opinions and expectations of others, I realized my self-worth. Gratitude is when you open your eyes to all of this and still feel blessed—for the good and the bad. It's saying thank you to a higher power for being exactly where you are and having what you have right now... no matter what destination lies ahead.

—Joel Relampagos, Executive Producer of NBC's:
The Biggest Loser and founder of *Change Your Algorithm*

Episode 17:

RADICAL GENEROSITY

My Dad often says, "It's nice to be nice, to people who are nice." (He is quite a philosopher.) But God calls us to be nice even when people aren't so nice. That is radical generosity.

Let me tell you, when you get a group of adults together, take away their vices, and then film them losing weight, they will inevitably become hungry and angry. We call them hangry! And when they are hangry, sometimes they won't be so nice. In those moments, I hope that what the contestants saw in me was radical generosity. It is what I strive for because I have experienced the healing power that it offers my soul and how highly contagious it can be.

Radical generosity isn't about how lavish a party you can throw for your friends, how much money you put in the basket on Sundays, how many boxes of Girl Scout cookies you buy to support the troops, or how many volunteer hours you donate. Radical generosity is about being kind when they don't deserve it, understanding when it doesn't make sense, fair even though you've been cheated, honest when you have been lied to, forgiving when it's unforgivable, and loving even when they are turning it away.

Give it to me straight

Through Christ's sacrifice, you have received all of those gifts and more. Now it's time to give them freely and in abundance because when you are generous with these gifts:

⊕ You will resemble Christ. Jesus models radical generosity in His thoughts, words, and actions, and when we follow His example, we start to look more and more like Him.

> *Bear one another's burdens, and so fulfill the law of Christ.*
> *—Galatians 6:2*

⊕ You will experience enhanced feelings of well-being and blessing. When you go beyond your own self-centered desires and self-interest to give to others, your soul will grow and heal.

> *Remembering the words of the Lord Jesus, how he said,*
> *"It is more blessed to give than to receive."*
> *—Acts 20:35*

⊕ God will delight in your generosity. When we resemble His Son by stepping out of ourselves to care for His earthly children, God celebrates and the heavens rejoice.

> *God loves a cheerful giver.*
> *—2 Corinthians 9:7*

Sonya is the poster girl for radical generosity, and when I opened her book, *44 Lessons From a Loser*, right there on the first page, she exemplified what it means to give without reservation. She dedicated her book as follows:

> *"This book is dedicated to you, the reader.*
> *The deepest desire of my heart is to pay forward all that I have learned from my time on The Biggest Loser."*

There is nothing that you will ever receive that will make you feel quite as good as if you had given it away. Get out there and start living a radically generous life; the health of your soul depends on it.

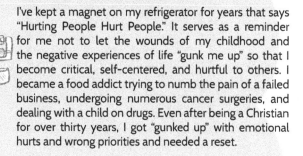

WEIGHING IN

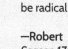

I've kept a magnet on my refrigerator for years that says "Hurting People Hurt People." It serves as a reminder for me not to let the wounds of my childhood and the negative experiences of life "gunk me up" so that I become critical, self-centered, and hurtful to others. I became a food addict trying to numb the pain of a failed business, undergoing numerous cancer surgeries, and dealing with a child on drugs. Even after being a Christian for over thirty years, I got "gunked up" with emotional hurts and wrong priorities and needed a reset.

The entire cast and crew of *The Biggest Loser* provided an environment of healing, both physically and emotionally. They helped with the physical pain of extreme workouts and spoke words of encouragement, hope, and praise to help un-gunk my soul. In wanting to repay that kindness, I pray almost every day now "Lord, show me someone to encourage and bless with my words, time, and resources," and He always leads me to someone. It's absolutely free to affirm someone with a word of praise or hope or to simply offer them your time. Radical generosity creates an advantageous environment and liberates a gunked-up soul for the spirit of Christ to come in and heal. Buy someone coffee or lunch and speak life into them. Be an encourager on social media where it's really easy to find someone that needs words of love and support. A Christ follower is called to be healed and to help others heal, to be radical in generosity

—**Robert Kidney** former contestant *The Biggest Loser: Season 17: Temptation Nation*

Episode 18:

ACCEPT GOD'S GRACE

When you are in a relationship with God, His plans for you are bigger and better than anything you could have planned yourself. You just need to be open to and accept the free and unmerited favor of God, which is simply His grace.

Sonya was an elementary school physical education teacher outside of Springfield, Illinois. She loved her students, her colleagues, and mostly her summers off. She liked her life just as it was. But God saw in Sonya a special gift—a gift that was buried far beneath a facade that the things of this world had created. So as God so often does, He set into motion a series of events that would allow Sonya to reveal this gift to the world so He could lead her to where He needed her special gift the most.

Sonya kept God at the forefront of everything in her life, and her weight-loss journey wasn't going to be any different. She says that God was very transparent about why He was sending her down this path. It was to show her that she was fearfully and wonderfully made, something she had forgotten over the years of struggling with her weight and food addiction. Remembering this saved her. You might think her intense workouts or the strict diet that she maintained for those six months were her reasons for achieving success, but I contend that it was the strength of her soul and her desire to honor and glorify God that propelled her past seventeen other contestants to the final three in line for the grand prize. God knew exactly where He needed her to be and where her gift would be noticed.

Sonya did not win the $250,000 grand prize that season, but it didn't matter, because that wasn't why God led her there. There was something much bigger waiting for her on the other side of the finale.

Your mission, should you choose to accept it...

When Sonya left the show, she was asked, as former contestants often are, to share her story in numerous public forums. That is where Sonya fell in love with the idea of public speaking. Now, this was a miracle in and of itself because Sonya had most of her life suffered from a severe speech impediment. However, if you only know Sonya from her appearance on the show, you might not have noticed her stutter because when the cameras turned on, her stutter disappeared. Gift of tongues? Sonya reminds me that "when He calls you, He equips you." Through her appearance on a highly-rated TV show and her newly found love of public speaking, she was able to reach even more people and share the love of Christ through her own weight-loss struggles and victories. She was able to share all she experienced to help others take a leap of faith to heal their body, mind, and soul, and she did it all using a platform that God had handcrafted just for her.

As you tell Jesus's story, you become Jesus's story.
—Pray As You Go app

Soon after her speaking career started, HSHS Medical Group, a Catholic health care organization, sought her out to be the face of their health and wellness program. I always told her that the Catholics were going to draft her; her prayer game was far too valuable to not have in our lineup. She spent four years in that position while successfully maintaining her weight. That's why it was an easy transition when she was laid off this past year due to COVID-19 to once again, with the prompting of the Holy Spirit, step outside of her comfort zone and build a business where she could pay forward all she has lived and learned. She is now the owner and coach of "Losin' It With Sonya Jones," a wellness clinic that focuses on losing weight and keeping it off through the healing of body, mind, and spirit. And if you are looking for another great read, her book, *44 Lessons From a Loser*, will have you laughing and crying from chapter to chapter.

Sonya had her spiritual house in order... but she needed physical healing before her special gift could be revealed. God led her on this journey so she could glorify Him and share the love of Christ with others who need the healing power He so freely gives when we are open and accepting of His grace.

The best-version-of-yourself will be faithful to purposes and gifts given to you by God.
—*Allen Hunt, Nine Words*

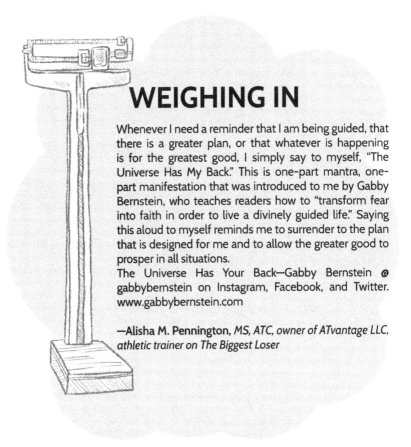

WEIGHING IN

Whenever I need a reminder that I am being guided, that there is a greater plan, or that whatever is happening is for the greatest good, I simply say to myself, "The Universe Has My Back." This is one-part mantra, one-part manifestation that was introduced to me by Gabby Bernstein, who teaches readers how to "transform fear into faith in order to live a divinely guided life." Saying this aloud to myself reminds me to surrender to the plan that is designed for me and to allow the greater good to prosper in all situations.

The Universe Has Your Back—Gabby Bernstein @ gabbybernstein on Instagram, Facebook, and Twitter. www.gabbybernstein.com

—**Alisha M. Pennington**, *MS, ATC, owner of ATvantage LLC, athletic trainer on The Biggest Loser*

SEASON FINALE:
SOUL

There you have it! Seven significant strategies to shepherd our souls and enable them to heal. We talked about being humble and allowing God to be in control. We discussed how prayer and silence can lead to great conversations with our Creator and how handing over our pain to Him can free us from the wounds we suffer. We saw that sacred moments, gratitude, and radical generosity all promote the magnification of our soul and help us to be more like Christ. And, finally, we learned that when our souls are prepared, the possibilities that God has in store for us are infinite.

Now let's put it all together and see what wellness actually looks like in the next season. But before we move on, answer this question truthfully.

Where is your soul broken, and what can you do to start the healing process today?

Season 5
WELLNESS

Colby's Story

The saints did not all begin well, but they all ended well.
—St. John Vianney

Colby's time on *The Biggest Loser* was spent in intense workouts and backbreaking self-discovery. Colby knew deep in his being that God had placed him on the show with purpose, but he spent months trying to figure out what that purpose could be. He would often say, "I know God put me here; I just gotta figure out why."

Colby was a hard-working young man from the Deep South that had been through several life-altering events: his father had committed suicide when Colby was only twenty-two years old, and a few years later, his brother was killed in a tragic car accident. It seemed like this young man couldn't take much more.

On a whim, a friend asked Colby to accompany him to *The Biggest Loser* audition as they were hosting an open casting call in the next town over. Colby hemmed and hawed and came up with every excuse in the book not to go, but with enough coaxing, he finally gave in and reluctantly agreed to tag along for the audition. And as happens in so many Hollywood stories, Colby made it through the first round of the casting cuts, but his friend did not. However, that season was a partner season, so the casting directors inquired if Colby had anyone to bring on as his partner. They asked if he had a father. Regrettably, Colby replied, "no sir." They asked if he had a brother, and again Colby sadly responded, "no sir." Then they asked, "Is there anyone you know that could be your partner on *The Biggest Loser*?" So Colby thought for a minute, perked up, then offered, "Well, I got me a pudgy wife!" The casting directors leaned in and asked, "How pudgy?"

Hope and Colby Wright were cast in season 17, Temptation Nation, and instantly became fan favorites during the first episode when the contestants were faced with a monetary temptation in exchange for their spot on the show. Colby justified his decision to pass up the money and stay on the ranch with his infamous line: "You can't buy thin!"

I don't know if it was his slow southern drawl or quick wit, but before long, Colby had exercised his way into viewers' hearts. Colby poured everything he had into each and every workout. It also didn't hurt that he was built like a mac truck and certainly wasn't afraid of a little hard work. He was losing weight, avoiding temptation, and getting stronger daily. And after a good long stint on the ranch, Colby headed home to Georgia to finish what he had started as one of the three finalists.

While he was at home competing for the grand prize of $250,000, an episode aired with Colby tearfully detailing how the numerous tragedies in his life had contributed to his excessive weight gain. Then Colby, uncomfortable and ashamed, recounted that one of the hardest days of his life was cleaning up after his daddy's suicide.

Soon after that episode aired, a viewer reached out to Colby to let him know how touched he had been by that story. He confessed that Colby's words had stopped him in his tracks and helped him to see how his own decisions would affect the lives of his family should he decide to go through with his plan to commit suicide. It was Colby's emotional and honest recollection of that night that changed the man's heart and saved his life.

Colby knew all along that God had a plan, bigger than anyone could have imagined. Colby had truly found the purpose he was so desperate to uncover through this journey. And there it was all spelled out for him. The purpose of his suffering, the meaning behind his pain, and the reason he was on the show.

By healing his body through leaving behind all of the bad habits and subsequently losing weight, addressing his mental health by learning to seek support and express his grief in a safe space, and most of all, by letting go of his pain, continuing to love the Lord, and trusting that God had a purpose for his life and the circumstances that brought him to *The Biggest Loser*, Colby won! No amount of money could have taken the place of the joy that filled his heart when he realized that God had kept His promise and used Colby's suffering to serve another in need.

When you have allowed the healing of your body, mind, and soul, God will use your story to glorify His name.

Today Colby and Hope are back home in Georgia. I used to tease them that if they hung around Los Angeles long enough, some big Hollywood producer would snap them up for a spin-off show called Somethin' Ain't Wright... with Hope and Colby.

Colby has returned to his love, announcing at the rodeo and working as a farrier shoeing horses. The two stay busy with the new additions to their family. They recently adopted a beautiful, cherub-faced little boy, and God then blessed them once again with a child of their own. Hope delivered their baby as I finished up this chapter, and we are reminded that God's timing is always perfect.

THAT'S A WRAP!

Well, my friends, here we are at the end of our time together. As I have written this guide to wellness, I have been on a journey myself. The beautiful memories that were stirred of people and places that I truly love offered me tears and laughter. The lessons that I learned gave me strength and the ability to move forward with this project. And the things that I lost along the way will never creep back into my life, including fear, procrastination, and doubt.

When God encouraged me to write this book, I thought it was to offer a road map of wellness for those who would someday pick it up and flip through its pages. But as God often does, He surprises us and reveals that we have been part of a much bigger plan all along, but we need to heal first. Writing this book offered me that healing. Sometimes you just need to get out of God's way, and He will do the rest. The things that I lost had been holding me back and not allowing me to learn what I needed to do in order to spread His grace and love.

I truly believe that God has a master plan for each of our lives, but we need to begin to heal our bodies, our minds, and our souls in order for that plan to be revealed to us. He needs us to be well in order to be effective disciples for Him. When you live in a state of wellness, you are changing not only yourself; you are changing the world forever. You will change your family, your future, and your legacy. And most importantly, you will change your relationship with God. And that, my friend, changes everything!

So ask yourself, What is getting in the way of being my very best me? And then take the advice of St. Francis of Assisi, who tells us to "start by doing what is necessary; then do what is possible; and suddenly you are doing the impossible."

Start your journey toward wellness today. I can guarantee that you will find the best you along the way, and that is when you will become the face of Christ for others.

I hope that you have also seen that *The Biggest Loser* was so much more than a weight-loss show, just like the story of the woman accused was so much more than a stranger happening upon a stoning. These were both events that changed the lives of the participants forever and deeply affected the hearts and minds of all those witnessing the healing of body, mind, and soul. If we want to transform the world, we have to be transformed first. Our God is the God of endurance and encouragement, and it is He who will give us the strength and courage to bear our crosses, face our demons, and transform the lives of many through our own stories of faith and renewal.

Instruction manual

> *Jesus bent down and wrote with his finger on the ground. And as they continued to ask him, he stood up and said to them, "Let him who is without sin among you be the first to throw a stone at her." And once more he bent down and wrote with his finger on the ground.*
> —*John 8: 6–8*

Through the centuries, there has been great conjecture as to what Jesus was writing on the ground that infamous day so long ago. Theologians speculate that He was writing the sins of the Pharisees and scribes which caused them to drop their stones and walk away. That idea sounds plausible. Historians theorize that He was fulfilling a prophecy from the Old Testament.

O LORD, the hope of Israel, all who forsake thee shall be put to shame; those who turn away from thee shall be written in the earth, for they have forsaken the LORD, the fountain of living water.
—Jeremiah 17: 13

It certainly wouldn't be the first time that happened! And still, others surmise that Jesus was simply doodling... a subtle shrugging off or cold shoulder to the Pharisees and their ridiculous attempt to trap Him yet again.

Now I am far from being a biblical scholar, but after the journey that we have been on together, I want to propose one more option. Maybe it's not too far-fetched to reason that when Jesus bent down and began to write in the sand that day, He knew that just like the woman, we would all come up against a time of healing and transformation at some point in our lives. So when He bent down to write in the sand, He was simply mapping out the instructions we would all need to care for His temples.

May God heal your body, mind, and soul so that you can ultimately experience wellness and with it, the fullness of life.

The glory of God is man fully alive.
—St. Irenaeus of Lyons

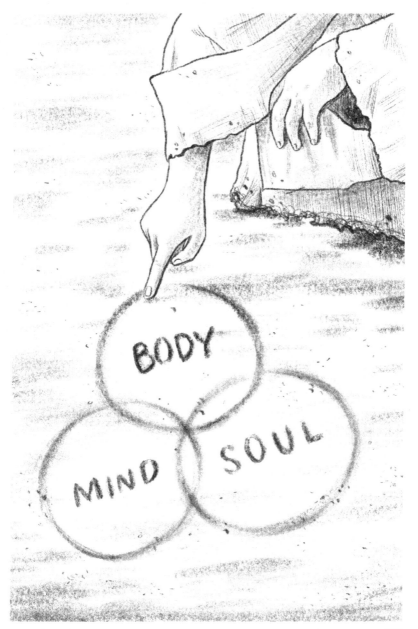

NOTES

[i] "What Is Wellness?" Global Wellness Day, February 11, 2017. https://www.globalwellnessday.org/about/what-is-wellness/.

[ii] "The Six Dimensions of Wellness." National Wellness Institute, accessed December 9, 2020. https://nationalwellness.org/resources/six-dimensions-of-wellness/.

[iii] "The Key to Creating Thriving Organizations." WELCOA, May 9, 2018. https://www.welcoa.org/blog/definition-of-wellness/.

[iv] "What Is Wellness?" Global Wellness Institute, May 14, 2019. https://globalwellnessinstitute.org/what-is-wellness/.

[v] "GWI Collaborates with the Vatican on 'Resetting the World with Wellness.'" Global Wellness Institute, May 20, 2020. https://globalwellnessinstitute.org/press-room/press-releases/the-vatican-taps-the-gwi-for-collaboration-on-resetting-the-world-with-wellness/.

[vi] West, Christopher. Theology of the Body for Beginners: Rediscovering the Meaning of Life, Love, Sex, and Gender. North Palm Beach, FL: Beacon Publishing, 2018.

[vii] Clark, Nancy. "Three Keys to Healthful Eating." In Nancy Clark's Sports Nutrition Guidebook, 6. Champaign, IL: Human Kinetics, 1990.

[viii] "5 Spices with Healthy Benefits." Johns Hopkins Medicine, accessed December 9, 2020. https://www.hopkinsmedicine.org/health/wellness-and-prevention/5-spices-with-healthy-benefits.

[ix] Sissons, Claire. "What Percentage of the Human Body Is Water?" Medical News Today. MediLexicon International, May 27, 2020. https://www.medicalnewstoday.com/articles/what-percentage-of-the-human-body-is-water.

[x] "Sugary Drinks." The Nutrition Source, October 16, 2019. https://www.hsph.harvard.edu/nutritionsource/healthy-drinks/sugary-drinks/.

[xi] Shortsleeve, Cassie. "How Sleep Can Affect Your Relationship, According to Science." Live Well. TIME, August 3, 2018. https://time.com/5348694/how-sleep-affects-relationships/.

[xii] "Are You Getting Enough Sleep?" Centers for Disease Control and Prevention, March 20, 2020. https://www.cdc.gov/sleep/features/getting-enough-sleep.html.

[xiii] Foster, Graham. "The Quotable Burgess." The International Anthony Burgess

Foundation, November 22, 2018. https://www.anthonyburgess.org/blog-posts/the-quotable-burgess/.

[xiv] "Depression and Anxiety: Exercise Eases Symptoms." Mayo Foundation for Medical Education and Research, September 27, 2017. https://www.mayoclinic.org/diseases-conditions/depression/in-depth/depression-and-exercise/art-20046495.

[xv] Merriam-Webster.com Dictionary, s.v. "mindfulness," accessed December 9, 2020, https://www.merriam-webster.com/dictionary/mindfulness.

[xvi] Touched By An Angel, Season 7 Episode 11, "The Hero," directed by Max Tash, aired January 7, 2001.

[xvii] Flippen, Flip, and Chris White. The Flip Side: Break Free of the Behaviors That Hold You Back. New York, NY: Springboard Press, 2008.

[xiii] Ackerman, Courtney E. "28 Benefits of Gratitude & Most Significant Research Findings." PositivePsychology.com, September 1, 2020. https://positivepsychology.com/benefits-gratitude-research-questions/.

[xix] Sansone, Randy A, and Lori A Sansone. "Gratitude and Well-Being: the Benefits of Appreciation." Psychiatry (Edgmont (Pa. : Township)) 7, no.11 (2010). https://www.ncbi.nlm.nih.gov/pmc/articles/PMC3010965/.

ACKNOWLEDGEMENTS

My God, with all my heart, thank you for answering my prayer so many years ago. I asked and you delivered. Please equip me with the courage to do the same, no matter what you ask of me.

I will never be able to fully express my gratitude to the fourteen "weighing-in" contributors. I am so honored that you agreed to be a part of my passion project, especially because this was a last-minute addition. Your words were uplifting, inspiring, full of heart, and in my inbox on time! I knew that each of you would nail it, and you did!

To all of the former contestants that allowed me to use their names and my own accounts of what happened, your candor and desire to share your journey is such a gift. I know that your beautiful stories will bring comfort and joy to those who need it most.

A huge thanks to all of the contestants that have passed through, and those that lived in, my training room. Your courage and determination have inspired this book. I wanted others to experience the pure joy you have brought to my life.

My husband and children supported me more than I could have imagined throughout this project. Brian, thank you for believing in me and cheering me on along the way. Maggie, thank you for tearing up each time I read you a chapter, helping me believe I had something special to share. Danny, thank you for answering all of my Google Doc questions and teaching me how to use a citation generator! It was life changing for me! And Mick, thank you for the comic relief when I was overcome with doubt and fear.

Shannon, my big sister, you are a poetic angel. Thank you for the beautiful book description and for knowing me well enough to nail the "about the author" page.

Kevin, my little brother, your time and insight was an answer to prayers. Thank you for allowing me to lean on you for support.

Marianne, my dear friend, thank you for being the first to read the book and decorate its pages with hearts and smiley faces! Your willingness to support and encourage me was priceless.

Thank you to my immediate and extended family for checking in on me throughout the writing process and encouraging me to complete this book in a timely fashion. I could feel your prayers lifting me up and carrying me forward while I was writing. I love you all so much and am exceptionally proud to call you my family.

A big thanks to the team at Self-Publishing School, especially my coaches. Gary, you truly are the Yoda of book writing! Ellaine, your insight and love of the Lord led me through the home stretch.

A special thank you to all those who said, "I can't wait to read your book." You are the reason it came to fruition. Your enthusiasm was contagious.

The woman accused. You are so much more than a Bible story to me. Thank you for allowing me to use your life as an example to help others heal through the intercessions of Christ. I pray that your soul rests with God, and I look forward to making your acquaintance when my journey is finished and I am welcomed home.

LOSING, LEARNING, AND LOVING

128

ABOUT THE AUTHOR

Kelly Hudson is proud to have served the men and women of the hit reality TV show *The Biggest Loser* as the head athletic trainer and director of sports medicine during the show's last three seasons. President of *ThAT's A Wrap Sports Medicine* and certified athletic trainer, Kelly specializes in the prevention, care, and rehabilitation of performance-related injuries. For over twenty-five years, she has worked globally with the talented performers of:

- The Radio City Rockettes ⊕ Michael Flatley's Lord of the Dance
- The Jabbawockeez Dance Crew
- Broadway's Burn the Floor: Ballroom. Reinvented

She is also known for her innovative development of professional performance medicine programs at:

- Disneyland Entertainment ⊕ Action Horizons Stunts
- The WaterWorld Stunt Show Spectacular

She is a popular speaker, engaging teenage and adult audiences with her unique brand of humor and faith-based content, including:

- "REALationships" Building Healthy Relationships
- Losing, Learning, and Loving
- Fully Engaged: With Family, The Mass, and Your Parish

Kelly Hudson is a Catholic ambassador who has a passion for helping others to see the presence of God in their lives. A native of Syracuse, New York, she now resides in Orange County, CA, with her incredibly talented husband and three young adult children, who keep her laughing and never cease to amaze her and God. They are collaborating on that project as well!

To contact her about potential speaking engagements, email her at: LosingLearningLoving@gmail.com

**I wouldn't truly be an Irish girl
If I didn't leave you with a wee limerick**

Thank you for reading my book!
I'm delighted you gave it a look.
And now that you're done,
The favor I'll ask is just one.
Can you help me create a hook?

All I'm asking you to do
is in a sentence, or two,
let me know what you thought,
if you enjoyed what you bought,
by leaving an honest review.

Slàinte Mhaith,
(Good Health)
Kelly

/